Health and Beauty Therapy

A Practical Approach for NVQ Level 3

Health and Beauty Therapy

A Practical Approach for NVQ Level 3

Dawn Mernagh
Jennifer Cartwright

Stanley Thornes (Publishers) Ltd

First published in 1995 by:
Stanley Thornes (Publishers) Ltd
Ellenborough House
Wellington Street
CHELTENHAM
GL50 1YW
United Kingdom

99 00 / 10 9 8 7 6 5 4

A catalogue record for this book is available from the British Library.

ISBN 0 7487 1817 6

Typeset by P&R Typesetters Ltd, Salisbury
Printed and bound in Great Britain by Redwood Books, Trowbridge, Wiltshire.

Contents

Acknowledgements

We wish to express our thanks to Ken Ward, David Cartwright and our families and friends for their support and encouragement whilst researching and writing this book.

Special thanks to: Rod and Angie Fabes (Carlton Professional), Vanessa Puttick (The Hairdressing and Beauty Equipment Centre), Richard Warden (Helionova), Sharon Williamson (The International Dermal Institute), Pam Baddesley, Val Cooke, Chris Elliot, Heather Lulham and Gaye Wensley for their technical assistance.

Acknowledgement and thanks are due to Janet Simms, author of A Practical Guide to Beauty Therapy for NVQ Level 2, for work reproduced in Chapters 3 and 11 of this book.

We are extremely grateful to our colleagues in the beauty industry, in particular the companies that have kindly allowed us to reproduce photographs and illustrations:

Cover photograph; Aromist, courtesy of Vanity Fayre Group.
Figures 4.7, 4.66, 5.8, 6.1, 6.11, 6.30, 7.5, 8.3, courtesy of Carlton Professional.
Figures 6.18, 7.6, courtesy of The Hairdressing and Beauty Equipment Centre Ltd.
Figure 3.2, courtesy of Prestige Medical.
Figure 3.7, courtesy of Leonard Drake salon, Los Angeles, USA.
Figures 10.1, 10.3, courtesy of Rita Roberts.
Figure 6.26, courtesy of Ultratone™ Bodyshapers.
Figure 7.1, courtesy of Middleton Leisure.
Figure 7.3, courtesy of Belle Santé (UK) Ltd.
Figure 7.4, courtesy of Laboratoires Guinot.
Figure 8.2, courtesy of Frevila Ltd.
Figure 9.6, courtesy of Helionova Ltd.
Figure 9.7, courtesy of Aim Beauty Complex, Bangkok, Thailand.
Figure 11.1, courtesy of Nu-Vogue, Leamington Spa.

Study Matrix for NVQ/SVQ units

Chapter	B04	B17	C01	C02	C03	C04	C05	C06	C07	C08	C09	C10
1			•			•	•	•	•	•		•
2			•			•	•	•	•			•
3	•	•	•	•	•	•	•	•	•	•	•	•
4			•			•						
5							•			•		•
6			•				•					
7												
8			•									•
9			•				•			•		
10			•								•	
11		•		•	•	•	•			•		•

NVQ/SVQ Level III Beauty

Core units*
B04* – Undertake salon reception duties
B17* – Handling stock (DOSC)
C01 – Assess the client for treatment
C02 – Maintain services and operations to meet quality standards (MC1)
C03 – Contribute to the planning, monitoring and control of resources (MC1)

Mandatory units
C04 – Provide body massage
C05 – Provide mechanical and electrical treatments for the head, neck, limbs and trunk
C06 – Provide advice on dietary control
C07 – Provide individual exercise

Additional Level III units
C08 – Provide sun-bed tanning treatment
C09 – Provide and instruct on remedial camouflage
C10 – Provide heat and bath treatment

*These units are transferable across levels.

Introduction

A career in beauty therapy has never been more exciting as technologies continue to advance to meet the growing demands of the public. It is however a very challenging profession due to the fact that by its nature it is a caring industry requiring a great deal of sympathy, empathy and understanding by the therapist. The range and breadth of the skills and knowledge covered are vast and it is essential that the therapist remembers that they will continue to learn new skills and further enhance existing ones throughout their career. Opportunities for the therapist expand every year, particularly as advancements in travel have made the world a much smaller place.

Health and Beauty Therapy: a Practical Approach for NVQ *Level* 3 is intended as a guide for trainees studying for NVQ/SVQ at level 3 in Beauty Therapy who have prior knowledge of anatomy, physiology and science. It is a useful reference book for beauty therapy examinations offered by BTEC, CIBTAC, CIDESCO, C & G, ITEC and VAI. It will also assist in updating qualified therapists, especially those who work on their own.

Wishing you success and happiness in your future careers

Dedication

This book is dedicated to Rod Fabes for his inspirational support and guidance to the beauty therapy industry.

Sadly Rod did not live to see publication of this book but his enthusiasm for our work and the education of future therapists remained to the end.

1 Anatomy and physiology

After working through this chapter you should:
> have a greater awareness of the structure and functions of the human body
> be able to give a brief outline of the structure and functions of the various systems of the body
> be able to relate this knowledge to the practical treatment situation where appropriate.

In order for the therapist to plan and perform effective treatment programmes for individual client's needs, it is essential to have an understanding of the structure and functions of the body. This chapter is designed to give an overview for therapists who have previous knowledge of anatomy and physiology and it is recommended that further study is undertaken from specialist sources.

Cells and tissues

The human body develops from a single cell called the *zygote* which results from the fusion of an *ovum* and *sperm*. Cell multiplication follows and as the foetus grows, cells with different structural and functional characteristics develop. However all cells carry the same genetic 'blueprint' as the initial zygote.

Structure of the cell

Fig. 1.1 *An animal cell*

All animal cells are composed of the following basic structures.

Cell membrane

This is really the cell wall and it keeps the cell contents intact. Substances can pass into and out of the cell across the membrane. It is a flexible structure and can change shape.

Cell fluid

Known as *cytoplasm*, cell fluid is a jelly-like substance that suspends all the cell's contents. Found within the cell fluid are folded membranes forming tubes known as *endoplasmic reticulum*, a structure which functions as a transportation channel.

In addition to the internal system of membranes there are other structures within the cytoplasm:

Mitochondria

Food substances such as sugar are broken down chemically in the mitochondria to release energy that is needed to drive the reactions in the cell.

Ribosomes

Ribosomes play a part in building up proteins from which all cells and tissues are constructed.

Golgi bodies

Golgi bodies are specialised structures found near the nucleus. Their main function is to add carbohydrate to cell protein.

Nucleus

The nucleus is the most important part of the cell. It is a large spherical body enclosed in a special cell fluid called protoplasm but separated from it by a nuclear membrane. In the nucleus there are a number of thread-like bodies called *chromosomes*. There are 46 chromosomes in every human cell which are arranged in pairs, one member from each pair being inherited from the male parent and the other from the female. The chromosomes contain the basic hereditary information which determines the individual's characteristics and traits, such as hair and eye colour, the structure of bones and teeth, etc.

---USEFUL INFORMATION---

Chromosomes are made of very long molecules of deoxyribonucleic acid (DNA).

Mitosis

Mitosis is the process of cell multiplication that occurs throughout life whereby cells are formed to replace those that have died. Mitosis is divided into four phases.

1 Prophase

A structure called a *centrosome* divides into two *centrioles* which migrate to opposite sides of the cell remaining attached by thread-like *spindles*.

2 Metaphase

The nuclear membrane disappears and the chromosomes arrange themselves at the centre of the cell. They are attached to the spindles of the centrioles.

Prophase

Metaphase

Anaphase   Telophase   Daughter cells

Fig. 1.2 *Cell division by mitosis*

3 Anaphase
The *centromere*, a structure that connects pairs of chromosomes, divides and the identical chromosomes move apart, breaking the spindle structure.

4 Telophase
The spindles disappear completely while the nuclear membrane reappears around each of the two groups of chromosomes. A constriction occurs around the middle of the cell body until eventually the cell divides into two. The two cells are known as *daughter cells*.

Types of tissues

Cells unite to form tissues within the body. There are four main types:

- Epithelial.
- Connective.
- Muscular.
- Nerve.

Epithelial tissue
This is the simplest form of tissue and consists of one layer of cells in the case of simple epithelium and two or more layers in the case of stratified

epithelium. This type of tissue forms the skin and is found within the linings of certain organs.

Connective tissue
There are many forms of connective tissue in the body. Adipose, bone and fibrous tissues are a few examples. Connective tissues can generally be thought of as tissue that unites other tissues together or gives support.

Muscular and nerve tissue
See pp. 14–20 for muscular tissue and pp. 28–31 for nerve tissue.

ACTIVITY

Research the different types of epithelial, connective, muscular and nerve tissue.

PROGRESS CHECK

1 Describe epithelial tissue.
2 Explain briefly the process of cell division by mitosis.

The skin

The human skin is the largest organ of the body covering an area of approximately 1.2–2 square metres. Its main purpose is one of protection. It keeps the internal structures of the body covered and intact and it has to be able to withstand daily wear and tear. It also protects the body against invasion by bacteria, chemicals and other foreign substances.

Fig. 1.3 *Vertical section of the skin*

The structure of the skin

Skin is composed of three main layers:

* Epidermis.
* Dermis.
* Subcutis.

Epidermis

This is the outer, visible layer of the skin and is itself composed of five distinctive layers. It takes approximately 30 days for this layer to renew itself and will vary in thickness on different parts of the body.

There are five distinct layers of the epidermis and these are:

1 Stratum germinativum (sometimes referred to as the basal layer). This is the deepest layer of the epidermis and consists of columnar cells which are mitotically active. The new cells produced by mitosis in the stratum germinativum are continually pushed up into the subsequent layers of the skin. *Melanocytes* are present within this layer and are responsible for producing the pigment *melanin*.

2 Stratum spinosum (sometimes referred to as the prickle cell layer). This layer is immediately above the basal layer and consists of cells with prickle-like projections which are connected to each other. They are living cells, each containing a nucleus.

3 Stratum granulosum. This layer is formed from rows of flattened cells which contain a granular protoplasm. The dark granules present are *keratohyaline* which is involved in the first stage of keratinisation.

4 Stratum lucidum. This layer consists of light-permeable, transparent cells which contain droplets of a substance called *eleidin*. Eleidin is formed from keratohyaline and transforms into *keratin*.

5 Stratum corneum. This is the visible layer of the epidermis. Its cells are completely flattened, keratinised structures with no nucleus. Cells are shed from the stratum corneum and replaced on a continuous basis. The stratum corneum usually consists of many flattened cells.

Fig. 1.4   *The layers of the epidermis*

Dermis

The dermis lies directly below the epidermis and is the thickest layer of the skin. It consists of two main layers known as the *superficial papillary layer* and the *reticular layer*. Found within the dermis are the following structures:

* **Collagen and elastin fibres.** Collagen is a protein constituent and is responsible for giving the skin its firm contours. Elastin is formed from connective tissue. The yellow elastin fibres give the skin its suppleness. Collagen and elastin both deteriorate with the natural ageing process.

* **Hair and hair follicles.** The hair follicle is a natural indentation within the dermis consisting of a downward extension of epidermal cells. The hair follicle is composed of an inner and outer root sheath which is surrounded by a connective tissue sheath. This sheath has a loosely-knit mesh of papillary cells overlying it, interspersed with nerves and blood capillaries. At the base of the follicle is a cluster of cells called the *dermal papilla* which provides the sole source of nourishment for the hair.

* **Sudoriferous glands.** These are found in abundance within the dermis and are composed of epithelial cells. They produce a watery substance known as sweat which travels via a duct to the surface of the skin through a pore, or otherwise open into hair follicles. There are two main types of sudoriferous gland; *eccrine glands* and *apocrine glands*. The latter glands do not become active until pubescence. Both play a part in the heat regulation of the body.

* **Sebaceous glands.** These are also found in abundance within the dermis and are composed of secretory epithelial cells. They produce a fatty substance called *sebum* and normally open into a hair follicle. Sebum keeps the hair lubricated and gives some protection to the surface of the skin.

* **Arrector pilorum muscles.** These are tiny, involuntary muscles attached to the hair follicle. The muscles respond to cold and fear causing them to contract and forcing the hairs within the follicles to stand on end, giving the skin the appearance of goose flesh.

* **Sensory nerve endings.** Within the dermis are nerve endings which respond to pain, pressure, heat, cold and touch. The nerves carry impulses to the brain. Without the responses made to impulses from the sensory nerve endings serious mechanical damage could occur to the skin and the body as a whole.

* **Lymph vessels.** These are found in abundance throughout the dermis. Lymph vessels help to drain excess fluid.

Subcutis

The subcutis is the third layer of the skin and is a type of connective tissue which divides the dermis from the muscular layer. It has a rich blood supply and contains some sensory nerve endings. The majority of the cells in this layer are fat cells which act as a buffer to prevent damage to the underlying structures and also insulate the body against heat loss. The thickness of the subcutis varies on different parts of the body, for example it is thicker on the gluteal area than the forehead. It is generally thicker on women than on men.

┌─ USEFUL INFORMATION ─┐

The hair is composed of three distinct layers; the cuticle layer, the cortex and the medulla.

6

Natural moisturising factor

The skin has a natural moisturising factor which is created within the cell regeneration and the production of the skin's acid mantle. It helps to prevent moisture loss from the epidermis. As the cells move upwards towards the surface of the skin, moisture is pushed from the inside of the cells outwards thus coating each cell with a sticky intercellular glue. This has the effect of holding the stratum corneum together.

The functions of the skin

The skin serves many important functions. The main ones are:

* **S**ecretion.
* **H**eat regulation.
* **A**bsorption.
* **P**rotection.
* **E**limination.
* **S**ensation.

Secretion

The two main substances the skin secretes are *sebum* and *sweat*.

Sebum is produced by the sebaceous glands which are situated in the dermis between the angle of the follicle and the arrector pilorum muscle. Sebum is a fatty substance which lubricates the skin's surface and the hair. Sebum is also bactericidal and so prevents bacterial infection.

Sweat is produced by the sudoriferous glands which are coiled tubules situated in the dermis. Sudoriferous glands open onto the skin's surface via a small duct (the sweat duct) and pore. There are two types of sweat gland:

* Eccrine glands are found in abundance all over the body. They secrete a clear, watery fluid.
* Apocrine glands are found under the arms (axillae) and in the groin area (inguinal). They produce a milky fluid. Apocrine glands start working from puberty onwards.

Heat regulation

Body temperature in good health is 36.9°C. For this temperature to remain constant a heat loss/production balance must be maintained. This is sometimes referred to as *homeostasis*.

Heat loss is affected by two main factors; the amount of blood circulating in the capillaries and the amount of sweat formed and its rate of evaporation.

Any increase in body temperature will have the following effects:

* *Vasodilation* occurs. The capillaries near the skin's surface dilate, allowing more blood to circulate nearer to the surface where heat will be lost by radiation and convection thus giving the skin a flushed look.
* Increased amounts of sweat are produced. This has a cooling effect as it evaporates from the surface of the skin.

USEFUL INFORMATION

Together, the sweat and sebum that mix on the surface of the skin form what is known as the acid mantle, *which, as the name suggests, is acidic and protects the skin from organism growth.*

A decrease in body temperature will have the opposite effects:

● *Vasoconstriction* occurs. Capillaries near the skin's surface constrict. Less blood flows near the surface and therefore less heat is lost.

● Sweat production diminishes.

Absorption

As one of the skin's main functions is to protect against the intrusion of foreign substances, the skin absorbs very little. Only tiny quantities of water and oil-soluble substances are absorbed.

However, the skin can be said to absorb radiation; in particular ultra-violet radiation. Ultra-violet rays penetrate the skin and act on a substance called *ergosterol* which is present in the subcutis of the skin, producing vitamin D.

Protection

The skin has several protection mechanisms:

● The stratum corneum (horny layer) of the epidermis contains keratinised cells which act as a buffer and are impervious to most substances.

● Sweat is acidic and has the effect of inhibiting organism growth.

● Sebum, as well as being bactericidal, acts as a lubricant preventing the surface of the skin from cracking. This also helps to prevent invasion by bacteria.

● Adipose tissue in the subcutis insulates the body and protects the underlying structures from bumps and knocks.

● Sensory nerve endings in the skin respond to painful stimuli to protect the body from mechanical and environmental damage.

● Melanin is produced in the skin in response to ultra-violet radiation. Certain types of ultra-violet radiation can cause damage to the skin, such as premature ageing and skin cancers. Melanin is produced to limit this damage.

Elimination

As has been previously mentioned the skin secretes sweat and sebum. These contain waste products that the body needs to eliminate.

Sensation

The sensory nerve endings found within the dermis protect the body from serious environmental and mechanical damage by reacting to pain, pressure, heat, cold, and touch.

USEFUL INFORMATION

Sweat contains: 99.4% water, 0.4% water-soluble substances such as urea and salt, 0.2% trace minerals and has a pH of 7.3.
Sebum contains: lipids (oils and fats – typically squalene, glycerol and cholesterol), carbohydrates and water and has a pH of 4.5.

pH of the skin

pH is the measurement of acidity or alkalinity. The pH scale ranges from 0–14 with 7 being neutral. The lower the number the more acidic and the higher the number the more alkaline. The skin has a pH between 4.5 and 6 making it acidic.

ACTIVITY   Describe the physiological effects of massage on the skin.

PROGRESS CHECK

1 Name the layers of the epidermis and give a brief description of each.

2 List the main functions of the skin.

The skeletal system

There are two types of skeleton;

1 Exoskeleton – this is where hard material is formed mainly on the outside of the body. Crustaceans normally have an exoskeleton.

2 Endoskeleton – this is where the skeleton is formed inside the soft tissue. The skeleton is made of bone and cartilage such as in human beings.

Functions of the skeleton

The skeleton has four main functions:

* Support.
* Protection.
* Muscle attachment.
* Movement (locomotion).

Support

The skeleton supports and raises the body from the ground and allows movement. Vital organs are suspended from the skeleton thus preventing them from crushing each other.

Protection

The skeleton is uniquely designed to protect the internal organs. In particular it protects:

* the brain, which is encased in the cranium
* the spinal cord, which is encased in the vertebral column
* the heart and lungs, which are surrounded by the rib cage.

The organs are protected by the skeleton from distortion resulting from pressure and from injury resulting from impact.

Muscle attachment

The skeleton acts as a framework for the voluntary muscular system. For movement to take place a muscle must be held in place firmly at one end (this is known as the origin of the muscle) and be free to move at the other end (this is known as the insertion of the muscle). The origins and insertions of most of the body's muscles are located on the bones of the skeleton.

Movement (locomotion)

Many bones of the skeleton act as levers. When muscles pull on these levers they produce movement, such as the chewing action of the jaw, the flexing of the biceps and the inhalation/exhalation movements of the ribs. All these movements require a system of joints and muscle attachments.

Frontal bone
Nasal bone
Sphenoid bone
Zygomatic bone
Maxilla (upper jawbone)
Mandible (lower jawbone)

Parietal bone
Occipital bone
Temporal bone
Cervical vertebrae (7)

Clavicle (collarbone)
Scapula (shoulder blade)
Sternum
Rib (12 pairs)
Thoracic vertebrae (12)
Humerus
Rib cartilage
Lumbar vertebrae (5)
Radius
Ulna
Ilium
Ischium
Pubis
Sacrum

Phalanges of the fingers
Carpal (wrist) bones   Metacarpal bones

Femur (thighbone)
Patella (knee cap)

Fibula
Tibia

Tarsal bones
Metatarsal bones
Phalanges of the toes

Fig. 1.5   *The skeleton*

Composition of the skeleton

The skeleton consists of some 204 bones in adult life.

* 22 form the cranium.
* 25 form the thorax.

10

* 33 form the spine.
* 120 form the upper and lower limbs.
* 4 form the pelvis.

Types of bone tissue

There are two types of bone tissue *compact* and *cancellous*.

Compact bone

Compact bone contains large numbers of structures called *Haversian systems*. An Haversian system consists of a central longitudinal canal, called the *Haversian canal*, rich in blood, lymph and nerves, surrounded by plates of bone arranged concentrically, called *lamellae*. Spaces between lamellae contain osteocytes or bone cells called *lucunae*. The Haversian systems are covered with a tough, fibrous sheeting called *periosteum*. This tubular formation makes this type of bone strong and rigid.

Cancellous bone

Cancellous bone appears more 'spongy' than compact bone. It has larger Haversian canals with less lamellae, giving a latticework appearance. Cancellous bone contains red bone marrow.

Periosteum

Periosteum is the fibrous sheeting which covers the bone surface. It is composed of two layers. The inner layer produces new cells for bone growth. The outer, fibrous layer has a rich vascular supply.

Classification of bones

Long bones

The strongest bones of the skeleton, long bones are composed of a shaft (diaphysis) and two ends (epiphyses). The diaphysis is formed from compact bone while the epiphyses have an outer covering of compact bone with cancellous bone found within. An example of a long bone is the femur.

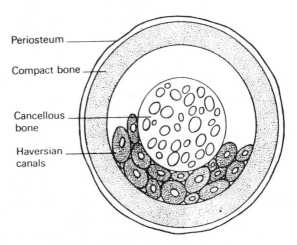

Periosteum

Compact bone

Cancellous bone

Haversian canals

Fig. 1.6 *Cross section through a long bone*

Short bones

Short bones are the small bones found in the wrists and ankles. They consist of a relatively thin outer layer of compact bone with cancellous bone inside. Examples of short bones are the metatarsals.

Flat bones

Flat bones consist of two thin layers of compact bone joined by a layer of cancellous bone and covered by periosteum. Two sets of blood vessels pass into the bone to supply the spongy and compact tissues. Examples of flat bones include the frontal and parietal bones of the cranium.

Irregular bones

Irregular bones consist of a mass of cancellous bone covered by a thin layer of compact bone overlaid with periosteum. Examples of irregular bones are the vertebrae.

Sesamoid bones

Sesamoid bones are rounded masses of bone tissue found in certain tendons. The best example of a sesamoid bone is the patella.

Joints

Where two or more bones come together a joint is formed. There are three main classifications of joint: *cartilaginous*, *fibrous* and *synovial*.

Cartilaginous joints are slightly moveable joints. They are held together by strong ligaments. The bones are separated by pads of white fibro-cartilage which allow only slight movement when the fibro-cartilage pad is compressed. Examples of this type of joint include the sacro-iliac joint and the symphysis pubis.

Fibrous joints are fixed joints. They do not allow any form of movement. Fibrous tissue is found between the bones in these joints. Examples of fibrous joints are the sutures between the bones of the skull.

Synovial joints are freely moveable joints. They allow a considerable amount of movement. The joint is enclosed in a fibrous capsule supported by ligaments. The capsule is lined by a synovial membrane which secretes synovial fluid into the capsule. Synovial fluid prevents friction between articulating surfaces of the joint which are both covered in hyaline cartilage for smooth operation.

The types of synovial joint are:

- Ball and socket joints.
- Hinge joints.
- Pivot articulations.
- Gliding joints.

Synovial joints are capable of the following types of movement:

a Extension – when a limb is extended, two parts of the limb are pulled away from each other (Fig. 1.7a).

b Flexion – when a limb is flexed, two parts of the limb are pulled towards each other (Fig. 1.7b).

a Extension   b Flexion   c Abduction   d Adduction

Fig. 1.7   *Movements of the upper limb*

Fig. 1.8   *Rotation*

c   Abduction – when a limb is pulled away from the midline (median line) of the body (Fig. 1.7c).

d   Adduction – when a limb is pulled towards the midline of the body (Fig. 1.7d).

e   Circumduction – combination of flexion, extension, abduction and adduction.

f   Rotation – movement round the long axis of bone (Fig. 1.8).

g   Pronation – when a limb is turned to face downwards.

h   Supination – when a limb is turned to face upwards.

i   Inversion – when a limb is turned to face inwards.

j   Eversion – when a limb is turned to face outwards.

Ball and socket joints

These joints are capable of flexion, extension, abduction, adduction, rotation and circumduction. Examples of ball and socket joints include the hip and shoulder.

Hinge joints

These joints allow for flexion and extension. Examples of hinge joints include the knee, elbow, ankle and the joint between the atlas and occipital bone in the head.

Pivot articulations

These joints allow for rotation only. Examples include the joint between the radius and ulna and the axis joint of the head.

Gliding joints

In these joints the articular surfaces glide over each other. Examples of gliding joints are the tarsal joint of the ankle and the carpal joint of the wrist.

ACTIVITY

With a colleague, undertake the following activities, noting which bones and types of joints are being used:

a walking up stairs
b catching a ball
c rotating the head.

PROGRESS CHECK

1 Give the functions of the skeleton.
2 Name two classifications of joints.

The muscular system

Roughly one fifth of body weight is that of muscle. It is muscle which forms the flesh of the body and moves, with the aid of the skeleton, the body. Whilst most muscles are attached to bones, there are exceptions, such as the epicranial aponeurosis. Both ends of the epicranial aponeurosis are attached to the skin. The muscle causes movements such as frowning, raising of the eyebrows, etc.

The naming of muscles is complicated. They can be named according to:

- Function, e.g. flexor or extensor, adductor or abductor, supinator or pronator.
- Attachments, e.g. sternocleidomastoid.
- Shape, e.g. trapezius.
- Formation, e.g. biceps (2 heads), triceps (3 heads), quadriceps (4 heads).
- Position, e.g. intercostal muscles (between the ribs).

USEFUL INFORMATION

The composition of muscular tissue is:
* *75% water.*
* *25% solids, of which the most important is a protein called myosin.*

Types of muscular tissue

There are three types of muscular tissue: *voluntary, involuntary* and *cardiac*.

Voluntary muscular tissue

Voluntary muscle is also called striated muscle and forms the flesh of the limbs and trunk. It consists of long fibres, made of multi-nucleate cells, which vary considerably in length according to the individual muscle. Each fibre contains numerous thread-like structures called *myofibrils*. Myofibrils are alternately striped in regular light and dark bands which is why voluntary muscle is sometimes called striated muscle. Muscle fibres are surrounded by a membrane called the *endomysium*. The fibres are bound together in bundles called *fasciculi* and surrounded by a sheath called the *perimysium*. The fasciculi in turn form a bigger bundle enclosed by a sheath called the *epimysium* which ultimately forms an individual muscle.

As the name suggests, voluntary muscle is under conscious control. It contracts quickly when stimulated by nerve impulses but tires rather quickly as well.

14

Trapezius

Deltoid

Triceps

Latissimus dorsi

External oblique

Gluteus maximus

Adductor magnus

Biceps femoris

Gastrocnemius

Tendon achilles

Erector spinae

Gracilis

Semitendinosus

Semimembranosus

Soleus

Fig. 1.9 *Muscles of the body — posterior view*

Involuntary muscular tissue

This type of muscle is found in the walls of the internal organs, e.g. stomach, bowel, uterus, etc. It consists of spindle-shaped cells, each of which contain a nucleus. These cells are unstriped and have no sheath but are bound together by connective tissue. They are not under control of will and are designed for slow contraction over a long period. Involuntary muscle, therefore, does not fatigue easily.

Sternocleidomastoid

Deltoid

Pectoralis major

Brachialis

Biceps

Serratus anterior

Internal oblique

Rectus abdominis

Tensor fascia latae

Sartorius

Rectus femoris

Vastus lateralis

Vastus medialis

Adductor brevis

Vastus intermedius

Adductor longus

Gracilis

Adductor magnus

Tibialis anterior

Fig. 1.10 *Muscles of the body — anterior view*

Cardiac muscle

This type of muscle is found only in the heart wall and is both involuntary and irregularly striped. It consists of short, cylindrical, branched fibres with a centrally placed nucleus. Cardiac muscle has no sheath but is bound together by connective tissue. It is not under control of will and contracts automatically throughout life in a rhythmical pattern. The rate of these contractions is controlled by nerves which quicken or slow down the action. This is the strongest type of muscular tissue within the human body.

The properties of muscular tissue

Muscle has four main properties:

* The power of contraction.
* Elasticity.
* Fatigue.
* Muscle tone.

The power of contraction

Voluntary muscle contracts as a result of stimuli reaching it from the nervous system and many nerves have their endings in muscles. Messages passing down a nerve from the brain cause the muscle to contract when they reach it. Other stimuli such as electrical currents applied directly to the muscle or its nerve will also cause contraction.

Elasticity and fatigue

When a muscle contracts, it uses energy which is derived mainly from the respiration of glucose. Glucose is supplied to the muscle via the blood. The blood also carries oxygen which the muscle uses to 'burn up' the glucose. During normal activity, the glucose is respired *aerobically*, that is the glucose is broken down to form water and carbon dioxide. The water and carbon dioxide are removed from the muscle and it does not tire.

During heavy exercise glucose is respired *anaerobically*. Anaerobic respiration produces *lactic acid* which is ultimately broken down to form carbon dioxide and water. However, lactic acid is not broken down very fast. After a certain number of contractions lactic acid begins to accumulate in the muscle. The muscle then becomes tired and is unable to contract with the same degree of efficiency. This affects the elasticity of the muscle and ultimately results in fatigue.

Muscular tone

Even when a muscle appears to be at rest it is always partially contracted and therefore ready for immediate action. This state of partial contraction is called muscular tone.

Tendons

Tendons are tough, fibrous and inelastic. They are found at the ends of muscles and their main purpose is to provide attachment to bones.

Ligaments

Like the tendons above, ligaments are strong, fibrous and do not stretch. Their function is to connect bones together.

ACTIVITY	Cut out pictures from magazines of people performing everyday activities such as cycling, walking, etc., then state which muscle or key muscle groups they are using.

Table 1.1 *The major muscles of the body*

	Position	Origin	Insertion	Action
Muscles of the neck and back				
Sternocleidomastoid	Front of the neck	Sternum and clavicle	Mastoid process	Used separately, turns the head to opposite side; used together, flexes the neck
Trapezius	Back of the neck and chest	Occiput and spines of the thoracic vertebrae	Spine of the scapula and clavicle	Draws scapula back, bracing the shoulders; pulls the occiput, extending the neck
Latissimus dorsi	Crosses the back from the lumbar region to the shoulder	Lumbar vertebrae, sacrum and back of iliac crest	Humerus	Adduction of the shoulder, drawing the arm back and downwards
Erector spinae	Between the tranverse and spinal processes of the vertebrae	Sacrum	Occipital bone	Keeps the body in an upright position and produces extension of of the vertebral column
Serratus anterior	Lateral chest wall	Upper nine ribs	Vertebral border of scapula	Draws shoulder forwards and rotates scapula
Muscles of the chest				
Pectoralis major	Front of the chest	Sternum and clavicle	Humerus, outer edge of the bicipital groove	Adduction of the shoulder, drawing the arm across the thorax
Muscles of the arm				
Biceps	Front of arm	By two heads from the scapula (coracoid process and above the glenoid cavity)	Radial tuberosity	Flexion of the elbow and shoulder; supinates hand
Triceps	Back of arm	By one head from the scapula and by two heads from the shaft of the humerus	Olecranon process of ulna	Extension of the elbow and shoulder
Deltoid	Over the shoulder	Spine of scapula and clavicle	Deltoid tubercle of humerus	Abducts the shoulder to a right angle
Brachialis	Crosses front of elbow	Humerus	Ulna	Flexion of the elbow

Table 1.1   *The major muscles of the body (continued)*

	Position	Origin	Insertion	Action
Muscles of the abdomen				
Rectus abdominis	Front of the abdominal wall	Upper border of pubic bone	5th, 6th and 7th costal cartilages and xiphoid process	Flexes the spine and aids respiration
External oblique	Forms the outer coat of the side abdominal wall	Lower ribs	Iliac crest	Flexes trunk together with internal oblique
Internal oblique	Forms the second coat of the side wall of the abdomen	Iliac crest	Lower ribs and fascia of the rectus abdominis	Flexes trunk together with external oblique. Produces rotation when used with the external oblique of the opposite side
Muscles of the buttocks				
Gluteus maximus	Large quadrilateral mass forming the prominence of the buttocks	Outer surface of ilium, also sacrum and coccyx	Upper end of femur	Extends the hip joint and rotates it laterally
Gluteus medius	Lies below the gluteus maximus	Gluteal surface of ilium	Greater trochanter of femur	Abduction of the hip joint
Muscles of the hip and upper leg				
Quadriceps	This extensive muscle mass forms the bulk of the anterior region of the thigh and is divided here into four separate muscles; the rectus femoris, vastus lateralis, vastus medialis and vastus intermedius			
Rectus femoris	Front of thigh	Ilium	Upper border of patella	Flexes the hip joint
Vastus lateralis	Lateral side of femur	Greater trochanter and linea aspera of femur	Tibial tubercle	Extends the knee joint
Vastus medialis	Medial side of femur	Lesser trochanter of femur	Tibial tubercle	Extends the knee joint
Vastus intermedius	Covers front of femur	Upper end of femur	Tibial tubercle	Extends the knee joint
Abductors of hip	Outer side of thigh	Anterior aspect of ilium	Between the two layers of a fascia lata	Abducts the hip

Table 1.1 *The major muscles of the body (continued)*

	Position	Origin	Insertion	Action
Muscles of the hip and upper leg (continued)				
Adductors of hip (pectineus, adductor brevis, adductor longus, adductor magnus, gracilis)	The group lies on the medial side of the thigh	Pubic bone	Linea aspera of femur	Adducts the femur
Hamstrings (biceps femoris, semimembranosus, semitendinosus)	Back of thigh	Ischial tuberosity and femur	Tibia and fibula	Extension of hip and flexion of knee
Sartorius	Crosses over the front of the thigh	Anterior superior iliac spine	Upper part of tibia	Weak flexor of both hip and knee joints
Tensor fascia latae	Lateral aspect of upper thigh	Outer part of iliac crest	Fascia latae	Abducts and rotates the femur and extends the knee
Muscles of the lower leg				
Tibialis anterior	Front of leg	Lateral surface of upper end of tibia	Medial cuneiform bone	Flexion and inversion of the foot
Gastrocnemius	Posterior calf area	Condyles of femur	Calcaneum	Flexes foot
Soleus	Posterior of calf area	Head and upper part of fibula and tibia	Calcaneum	Flexes foot

PROGRESS CHECK

1 Draw and label diagrams of the main muscles of the body.
2 State the four properties of muscular tissue.

The circulatory system

The circulatory system consists of:

- Heart.
- Blood.
- Blood vessels.
- Lymph.
- Lymph vessels.

The heart

The heart is a hollow organ with walls made of cardiac muscle. It is approximately 10 cm long and weighs about 225 g in women and 240 g in

Fig. 1.11 *The heart*

men. The heart is situated in the thoracic cavity protected by the rib cage and it lies obliquely to the left hand side.

The heart is composed of three distinct layers:

1 Pericardium. This is a smooth, membranous covering which is formed of an outer fibrous layer and an inner, serous coat. Between these layers a serous fluid is secreted which allows for ease of movement between the two layers.

2 Myocardium. This is the muscular layer of the heart and is formed of a specialised, involuntary muscular tissue. This cardiac muscle is exceptionally strong. The fibres are bonded together in branches and it has to be able to contract rhythmically throughout life.

3 Endocardium. This is the inner, lining membrane of the myocardium layer. It is very thin and consists of flattened epithelial cells.

Internal structure of the heart
The heart is divided into a right and left side with a layer of myocardium called the *septum* separating them. Each side is divided into two chambers. There are four chambers in total; the right and left *atria* and the right and left *ventricles*. Valves separate the chambers on each side of the heart from each other. The valve separating the right atrium and ventricle is called the *tricuspid valve*. The valve separating the left atrium and ventricle is called the *bicuspid* or *mitral valve*. These valves open and close when the pressure changes within the chambers.

When cardiac muscle contracts it squeezes blood out of the heart and into the arteries which carry it to all parts of the body. When cardiac muscle relaxes the heart fills with blood from the veins. This mechanism of contraction and relaxation is known as the heart beat.

USEFUL INFORMATION

At rest the heart beats approximately 60 to 70 times a minute. During this time it pumps approximately five litres of blood around the body.

Flow of blood through the heart

Deoxygenated blood returns from the body to the right atrium of the heart via the largest veins of the body, the superior and inferior vena cavae. This blood is then squeezed through the tricuspid valve into the right ventricle from where it is then forced through the pulmonary artery which carries the deoxygenated blood to the lungs. Gaseous exchange takes place between the blood and the air in the lungs; carbon dioxide is excreted and oxygen is absorbed. The now oxygenated blood returns to the heart via the pulmonary veins which empty the blood into the left atrium. It passes through the bicuspid valve and into the left ventricle, then is forced into the largest artery of the body, the aorta, which carries the oxygenated blood to the rest of the body.

POINTS TO NOTE ▷

- *Veins carry blood towards the heart. They normally carry deoxygenated blood. However, the one exception to this is the pulmonary vein which carries oxygenated blood from the lungs to the heart.*

- *Arteries carry blood away from the heart. They normally carry oxygenated blood. However, the one exception to this is the pulmonary artery which carries deoxygenated blood from the heart to the lungs.*

- *The left side of the heart is slightly more muscular. This is to enable it to force blood out to all parts of the body via the aorta.*

Cardiac cycle

The contraction and relaxation of the heart is called the cardiac cycle and is divided into two phases:

1 Diastole – when blood is passing from the veins into the atria and then into the ventricles. Heart muscle is relaxed.

2 Systole – when the ventricles contract during systole the valves in the heart are pushed closed causing the pressure in the arteries to increase. This gives the pulse.

Blood

Blood consists of:

- Erythrocytes (red blood cells).
- Leucocytes (white blood cells).
- Platelets.
- Plasma.

Erythrocytes (red blood cells)

Erythrocytes are minute, biconcave discs made from spongy cytoplasm surrounded by an elastic membrane. Their red colour comes from haemoglobin combined with oxygen. *Haemoglobin* is a protein which contains iron and has a natural affinity with oxygen. Haemoglobin combines with oxygen to form *oxyhaemoglobin*. Red blood cells are the mechanism by which oxygen is transported around the body. Red blood

Cross section

Top view

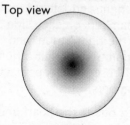

Biconcave disk

Fig. 1.12 *Erythrocyte (red blood cell)*

cells are made in red bone marrow. Cell formation takes approximately seven days, during which time the nucleus disappears and they cease to be true cells. The life span of a red blood cell is roughly four months, after which time the cell is destroyed in the liver or the spleen.

Leucocytes (white blood cells)

Leucocytes are colourless cells each containing a nucleus. There are far fewer white cells than red cells; approximately one to every six hundred red cells. The main function of white cells is to fight infection and protect the body against viruses, toxins and bacteria.

There are different types of leucocytes and they have different functions within the body.

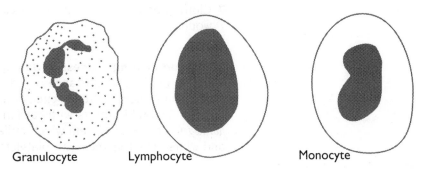

Granulocyte   Lymphocyte   Monocyte

Fig. 1.13   *Leucocytes (white blood cells)*

Granulocytes form approximately 75% of the total number of white cells. They ingest bacteria by encapsulating them and digesting them slowly – a process called phagocytosis. Granulocytes have a life span of about one week and are made in bone marrow.

Lymphocytes form roughly 23% of the total number of white cells. They are formed in lymph nodes and produce antibodies which kill foreign proteins. They can live for up to one hundred days.

Monocytes form approximately 2% of white cells. They can ingest foreign proteins in the blood.

Platelets

Platelets are formed in the red bone marrow and are fragments of red blood cells. They play an important part in the clotting process of blood.

Plasma

Plasma is a slightly alkaline, yellowish fluid in which the blood cells float. It consists of 96% water together with other important compounds such as:

- Proteins, e.g. albumen, fibrinogen, globulin.
- Antibodies.
- Soluble salts, e.g. sodium chloride, potassium chloride, calcium phosphate.

* Food substances, e.g. amino acids, glucose, fatty acids, glycerol.
* Waste products, e.g. urea, carbon dioxide.
* Hormones.

Functions of blood

1 Transport of oxygen from the lungs to the body tissues.
2 Transport of carbon dioxide from the body tissues to the lungs.
3 Transport of excretory products.
4 Transport of digested food.
5 Distribution of hormones.
6 Distribution of heat.
7 Clotting process of blood (this occurs to prevent loss of blood from a wound).

The blood clotting process in damaged tissue

Platelets produce a substance called *thrombokinase* which acts on *prothrombin* (which is already circulating in the blood) to change it to *thrombin*. Thrombin reacts with calcium ions in the blood producing *fibrinogen* – fibres of protein which radiate across the wound tangling red and white cells together with platelets – thus preventing blood loss.

Arteries and veins

Arteries and veins are hollow elastic tubes that transport blood which has been pumped by the heart around the body. They differ slightly in structure.

Fig. 1.14 *Cross sections of an artery and a vein*

Veins:

* have thinner walls than arteries
* contain valves to prevent the back-flow of blood
* carry deoxygenated blood (with the exception of the pulmonary vein mentioned earlier)
* have walls consisting of three layers – the tunica adventia, tunica media and tunica intima.

Arteries:

* have thicker walls than veins
* do not contain valves
* carry oxygenated blood (with the exception of the pulmonary artery mentioned earlier)
* have walls consisting of the same three layers as veins, but they are thicker than in veins.

Blood pressure

Blood pressure is the amount of pressure exerted on the arteries by blood as it flows through them. It is measured in millimetres of mercury (mmHg) using a *sphygmomanometer*.

The lymphatic system

The lymphatic system is a subsidiary or second circulatory system which drains the tissue fluid. It consists of a series of fluid-filled tubes beginning as fine, blind-ended capillaries which spread throughout most of the tissues of the body. These pass into larger lymphatic vessels which eventually drain into the great veins of the neck. The principal function of the lymphatic system is to fight infection within the body.

Lymphatic fluid

Lymph is a clear, straw-coloured liquid with a similar composition to blood plasma. Its main composition is water with some proteins, fats, hormones and salts. It contains white cells, mainly lymphocytes, together with waste products that the system is dealing with at any particular time, e.g. dead cells, micro-organisms.

Formation of lymph

Lymph is formed in the tissues of the body and is a derivative of blood plasma which passes out of the capillaries to form what is called intercellular fluid. Excess intercellular fluid drains into the lymphatic capillaries where it is known as lymph.

Lymphatic capillaries

Lymphatic capillaries are fine, hollow, blind-ended, elastic tubes, similar to blood capillaries in structure although they are wider and less regular in shape. They consist of a single layer of epithelial tissue, i.e. their walls are one cell thick, bound together with connective tissue. Because of this they are more permeable than blood capillaries, allowing for larger substances to pass through their walls. Lymph drains into them from the tissue fluids.

Lymphatic vessels

Lymphatic vessels carry lymph from the lymphatic capillaries to the great veins of the neck. They are composed of connective tissue lined with epithelial cells and they also contain valves to prevent back-flow to ensure that lymph flows away from the tissues.

Lymph nodes

Before lymph is discharged into the bloodstream it passes through at least one lymph node. Lymph nodes are situated in clusters around the

Fig. 1.15 *Cross section of a lymph node*

body and are composed of special cells which include *macrophages* which are phagocytic, i.e. they ingest foreign particles thereby filtering the lymph of toxins. Major groups of lymph nodes are in the head and neck, under the arms (axillae), in the breast area, abdomen and groin (inguinal). When there is localised infection within the body the lymph nodes in that particular area will become swollen as they are engorged with toxins.

The great veins of the neck

As has been mentioned previously, lymph travels through at least one lymph node before it returns to the blood stream. The vessels which allow lymph to re-enter the blood stream are called:

● **The right lymphatic duct.** This is a dilated vessel situated at the base of the neck and feeds into the right subclavian vein. It drains lymph from the right half of the head, neck, chest area and right arm.

● **The thoracic duct.** This vessel begins at the *cisterna chyli*, a specialised lymph sac found in front of the first two lumber vertebrae. It connects into the left subclavian vein at the base of the neck. It drains lymph from the left side of the head and neck, the left arm, left side of the chest area and both legs.

The spleen

The spleen is a large nodule of lymphoid tissue which is a deep purplish-red in colour. It is situated high up at the back of the abdomen on the left side behind the stomach. The functions of the spleen are:

● Formation of lymphocytes.

● A reservoir for blood.

● Formation of antibodies and antitoxins.

● Destruction of worn-out erythrocytes.

ACTIVITY	Research the ABO system of blood grouping.

PROGRESS CHECK	1 Name and describe the principle cells of the circulatory system.
	2 Describe the flow of blood through the heart.
	3 What is the main function of the lymphatic system?

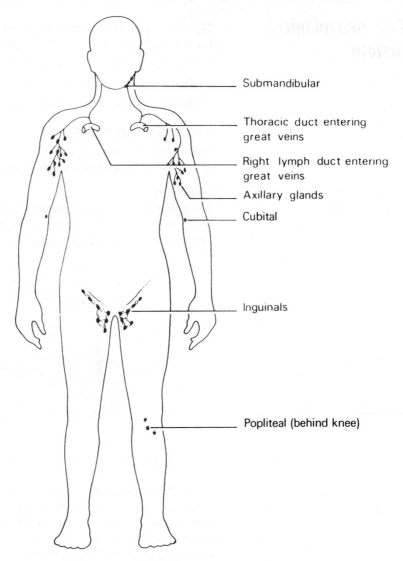

Fig. 1.16 *Lymph nodes of the body*

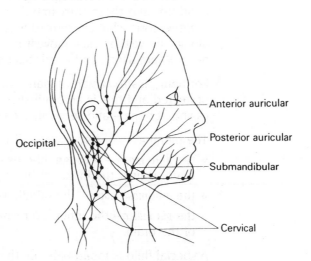

Fig. 1.17 *Lymph nodes of the face*

The neurological system

The neurological system is involved in transmitting messages from the brain to all other parts of the body. It consists of three main divisions:

1 The central nervous system.
2 The peripheral nervous system.
3 The autonomic nervous system.

The central nervous system

The central nervous system consists of the brain and spinal column and is at the centre of the neurological system.

The brain

The brain is the most important part of the entire neurological system. It receives impulses and stores them, it also transmits impulses to all parts of the body to stimulate organs to work.

Fig. 1.18   *Cross section through the brain*

The adult brain weighs approximately 1.5 kg and contains millions of neurones. Each neurone is composed of a cell body that is similar in composition to other animal cells in that it contains a nucleus and is surrounded by cytoplasm. However it differs in that it has a long tail known as its axon. The purpose of which is to control impulses away from the cell body. Attached to the cell body are small fibres called dendrites and these carry impulses into the cell. Groups of neurones together form what are termed nerves and in order for impulses to travel along a nerve they must move from the axon of one to the dendrite of the next. Where axons and dendrites meet is called the synapse.

For neurones to remain undamaged in the brain they need to be well protected and this is accomplished firstly by the skull – a hard outer casing of bone – and secondly by a specialised layer called the *meninges*.

The meninges consist of three distinct layers. These are:

- the *dura mater* – a tough, fibrous outer membrane which cushions the brain against the inside of the cranium
- the *arachnoid mater* – the middle layer, which is much more delicate
- the *pia mater* – the inner layer which folds into the convoluted surface of the brain.

A special fluid is found between the arachnoid and pia mater which acts as a further cushion. It is called *cerebrospinal fluid*.

The brain has three main regions: the *cerebrum, cerebellum* and *medulla oblongata*.

1 Cerebrum. The largest region of the brain, it is a dome-shaped area of nervous tissue split into two halves called cerebral hemispheres. The surface of the cerebrum is made of what is termed grey matter – this is where the main functions of the cerebrum are carried out. These functions include all forms of conscious activity. Sensations such as touch, vision, taste, hearing and smell originate here. Control of voluntary muscular movements and emotion, powers of reasoning and memory are also handled in the cerebrum.

2 Cerebellum. This region of the brain receives impulses from the semi-circular canals in the ears and from stretch receptors in the muscles. It processes this information to maintain muscle tone and a balanced posture. It also co-ordinates muscles during activities such as walking, running, dancing, etc.

3 Medulla oblongata. This region is often referred to as the *brain stem* and contains a mass of grey matter known as the *vital centre*. It controls the part of the nervous system not under control of will, e.g. regulation of blood pressure, body temperature, etc. It performs these functions through connections with the autonomic nervous system. The medulla oblongata also contains nerve fibres which connect the brain with the spinal cord.

The spinal cord
As mentioned, the spinal cord is continuous with the medulla oblongata and extends downwards through the vertebral column finishing at the level of the lumbar vertebrae. It is protected by meninges and cerebrospinal fluid like the brain. Radiating from the spinal column are 12

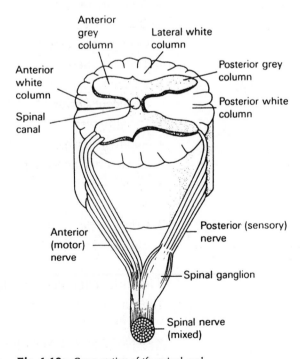

Fig. 1.19 *Cross section of the spinal cord*

pairs of cranial nerves and 31 pairs of spinal nerves corresponding to the segments of the vertebral column. The cranial and spinal nerves are part of the peripheral nervous system.

The peripheral nervous system

This part of the neurological system consists of all the nerves situated outside the central nervous system.

There are three types of nerve cell in the peripheral nervous system:

1 Motor (efferent) nerves. These nerves convey impulses from the brain through the spinal cord to the skeletal muscles, glands and smooth muscular tissue (effector organs).

2 Sensory (afferent) nerves. This type of nerve conveys impulses from the sensory nerves endings in organs to the brain and spinal cord.

3 Mixed nerves. These consist of both motor and sensory nerve fibres.

The peripheral nervous system consists of 31 pairs of spinal nerves and 12 pairs of cranial nerves.

The spinal nerves are as follows:

* 8 pairs cervical.
* 12 pairs thoracic.
* 5 pairs lumbar.
* 5 pairs sacral.
* 1 pair coccygeal.

The twelve pairs of cranial nerves are the:

* Olfactory nerves.
* Optic nerves.
* Oculomotor nerves.
* Trochlear nerves.
* Trigeminal nerves.
* Abducent nerves.
* Facial nerves.
* Auditory nerves.
* Glossopharyngeal nerves.
* Vagus nerves.
* Accessory nerves
* Hypoglossal nerves.

The autonomic nervous system

The autonomic division of the nervous system controls areas of the body over which there is no conscious control. It is divided into two sections:

* the sympathetic system
* the parasympathetic system.

The sympathetic system

The sympathetic system is composed of a gangliated cord which is situated on either side of the anterior surface of the vertebral column. It is composed of a network of interlaced nerves termed *plexuses*. The main plexuses of the sympathetic division are:

- solar plexus – which supplies the abdominal viscera
- cardiac plexus – which supplies the thoracic viscera
- hypogastric plexus – which supplies the pelvic region.

The parasympathetic system

This division is composed mainly of the vagus nerve which has the largest distribution of all the cranial nerves. It starts from nerve cells in the medulla oblongata and passes through the neck into the thorax and abdomen.

All the internal organs have in effect a double nerve supply, one supply from the sympathetic system and one from the parasympathetic system. The two systems work antagonistically. The sympathetic system increases body activity and the parasympathetic system slows it down.

The other area that the autonomic nervous system is involved with is the *reflex action*. This is an involuntary action designed to protect the body against serious damage. A very good example of this is if you touch a hot surface, before you have had time to register the pain in the normal way the reflex action spontaneously removes the finger.

ACTIVITY

Research the nerve supply for each of the muscles listed in this chapter.

PROGRESS CHECK

1 Name and describe briefly the main divisions of the neurological system.
2 List the spinal nerves.

The endocrine system

The endocrine, or hormonal, system is a series of ductless glands that secrete *hormones* (chemical messengers) which act on parts of the body other than where they were produced. Hormones are carried in the blood stream and influence many activities of the body.

The main endocrine glands of the body are:

- Pituitary gland.
- Thyroid gland.
- Parathyroid glands.
- Adrenal glands.

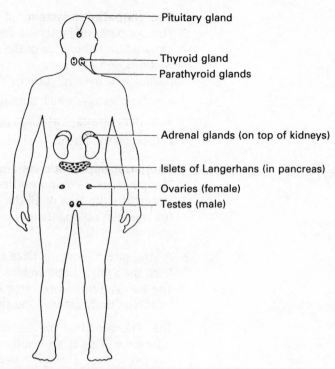

Fig. 1.20 *The endocrine glands*

- Pancreas – the islets of Langerhans.
- Ovaries (female only).
- Testes (male only).

The pituitary gland

The pituitary gland is sometimes referred to as the master gland because all the hormones it secretes have a bearing on all the other glands in the system. It is situated in the head in the hypophyseal fossa of the sphenoid bone below the hypothalamus to which it is attached by a isthmus. The gland consist of a posterior and anterior lobe.

Anterior lobe

The anterior lobe of the pituitary gland secretes eight hormones in total all controlled by what is termed *the negative feedback mechanism*. This means that when the level of any particular hormone is low in the blood supplying the hypothalamus, it stimulates the anterior lobe of the pituitary to produce the appropriate releasing hormone which stimulates the target endocrine gland that produces that hormone to produce more.

The eight hormones secreted by the anterior lobe of the pituitary and their functions are:

- Adrenocorticothrophic hormone (ACTH) – stimulates the adrenal cortex to secrete cortisol.
- Thyroid stimulating hormone (TSH)– stimulates activity and growth of the thyroid gland.
- Prolactin – directly affects the female breast immediately after childbirth to initiate and maintain milk secretion.

- Follicle stimulating hormone (FSH) – controls the maturation of the Graafian follicle in the ovary.
- Luteinising hormone (LH) – controls the activity of the gonads.
- Melanocyte stimulating hormone (MSH) – stimulates the production of melanin within the skin.
- Samatotrophin (HGH) – also known as human growth hormone, it promotes protein synthesis in growth and repair of all tissues.
- Interstitial cell stimulating hormone (ICSH) – controls gonad activity.

Posterior lobe

The posterior lobe of the pituitary gland secretes two hormones; *oxytocin* and *anti-diuretic hormone.*

Oxytocin promotes contraction of the uterine muscle and stimulates cells in the lactating breast to squeeze milk into the large ducts behind the nipple.

Anti-diuretic hormone (ADH) has two main functions:

- The *anti-diuretic effect* prevents water being lost from the kidneys and is influenced by osmotic pressure of the circulating blood.
- In large quantities ADH stimulates contraction of smooth muscle, especially in blood vessel walls, raising the blood pressure. This is called the *pressor effect.*

The thyroid gland

Situated in the lower part of the neck, the thyroid consists of a right and left lobe that lie either side of the trachea connected by an isthmus.

The thyroid secretes two main hormones:

- Thyroxin – necessary for controlling the metabolic rate, growth and differentiation of tissues, mental functioning and skin and hair condition.
- Calcitonin – reduces blood calcium levels by inhibiting the absorption of calcium from bones.

Parathyroid glands

The parathyroid glands are four small glands, two embedded in the posterior surface of each lobe of the thyroid gland. They secrete the hormone called *parathormone* which maintains the blood calcium concentration within its normal limits. It works in conjunction with calcitonin to control blood calcium levels.

Adrenal glands

There are two adrenal glands, one situated on the upper aspect of each kidney enclosed within the renal fascia. The glands are composed of two distinctive layers; the *adrenal cortex* and the *adrenal medulla.*

Adrenal cortex

The adrenal cortex produces three groups of hormones:

- Glucocorticoids – hormones which affect the regulation of carbohydrate metabolism, as well as helping in the formation of liver glycogen and helping *gluconeogenesis* (raising blood sugar levels). They suppress the body's inflammatory and allergic reactions and are connected with sodium and water reabsorption from the renal tubules.

* Mineral corticoids – hormones associated with the maintenance of the electrolyte balance in the body. They stimulate the reabsorption of sodium by the kidneys.
* Gonadocorticoids – sex hormones. The gonadocorticoids are *androgens* (male sex hormones) and the adrenal production is of little importance compared to the production of sex hormones by the ovaries/testes.

Adrenal medulla

The adrenal medulla is completely surrounded by the cortex, it is an extension of tissue from the same source as the nervous system and is closely linked to the sympathetic part of the autonomic nervous system.

The adrenal medulla secretes two hormones:

* Adrenaline (epinephrine) – associated with conditions needed for 'fight or flight'. Readies the body for immediate action. It triggers the constriction of peripheral blood vessels and the dilation of muscle fibres, enabling energy (food and oxygen) to be channelled where it is most needed. It also accelerates the conversion of glycogen to glucose.
* Noradrenaline (norepinephrine) – causes vasoconstriction and raises both systolic and diastolic blood pressure.

The pancreas

Hormones are produced in the pancreas by clusters of cells called *islets of Langerhans* which are distributed irregularly throughout the organ. There are three main types of cell in the islets of Langerhans. One of these cell types, the B cells, secrete the hormone *insulin* which together with glucagon, affects the level of glucose in the blood. The effect of insulin balances the effect of glucagon. Glucagon raises blood sugar levels while insulin reduces it.

The ovaries

The ovaries are the female gonads or sex glands. They are situated in shallow depressions on the lateral walls of the pelvis. The ovaries consist of a cortex and a medulla.

The ovarian cortex surrounds the medulla and contains ovarian follicles each of which contains an ovum. Throughout the reproductive years, one ovarian follicle matures, ruptures and releases its ovum during each menstrual cycle.

The ovarian medulla lies in the centre of the ovary and consists of fibrous tissue, blood vessels and nerves.

The two main hormones produced by the ovaries are:

* Oestrogen – influences the menstrual cycle. It stimulates the uterine lining to thicken to prepare for implantation should fertilisation occur.

It is also partly responsible for breast development – the growth of milk ducts in the breast. It also influences health and growth of bones, subcutaneous fat distribution and skin condition.

* Progesterone – connected with the development of the placenta and the maintenance of pregnancy when it occurs. It also prepares the mammary glands for lactation.

ACTIVITY   Research the effects of pregnancy on the female body.

The testes

The testes are the male gonads. They consist of 200 to 300 lobules composed of germinal epithelial cells. In-between these lobules are interstitial cells that secrete the main male hormone *testosterone*.

Testosterone is responsible for the secondary sexual characteristics that occur at puberty in males. Secondary sexual characteristics in males include:

* Increase in body hair.
* Deepening of the voice.
* Broadening of muscles.

PROGRESS CHECK   1 State the importance of the endocrine system.
                       2 Research the main disorders of the endocrine system.

The respiratory system

The respiratory system is involved in the taking in of oxygen and the removal of carbon dioxide from the body. This process is achieved through a number of specialised organs and tissues.

The respiratory system consists of:

* Nose.
* Pharynx.
* Larynx.
* Trachea.
* Two bronchi.
* Bronchioles.
* Two lungs.
* Intercostal muscles.
* Diaphragm.

Nose

The function of the nose is to warm, filter and moisten air. This function is achieved by tiny, ciliated, columnar epithelium which trap bacteria and

35

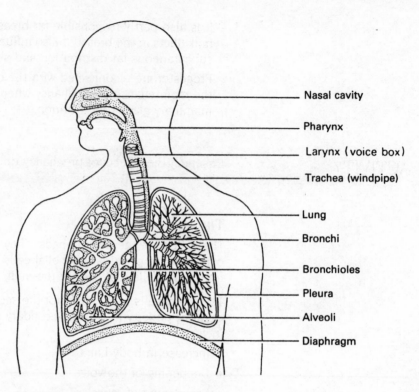

Fig. 1.21 *The respiratory system*

dust. They secrete mucous which moistens the air as well as acting as an adhesive medium to prevent bacteria and dust entering the throat. Once air has passed through the nose it moves on to the pharynx.

Pharynx

The pharynx has both a respiratory and a digestive function. The respiratory function of the pharynx is similar to that of the nose – it further warms and moistens air before it travels on to the next air passage, called the larynx.

Larynx

At the top of the larynx there is a flap of tissue called the *epiglottis* which closes to stop food entering the trachea during swallowing. Air passing over the vocal cords within the larynx produces the voice.

Trachea

Also referred to as the windpipe, the trachea consists of a tube surrounded by c-shaped rings of cartilage that act to keep the trachea open even when the neck is bent. It is lined with ciliated epithelium which secrete mucous – a further air-filtration system.

Bronchi

There are two bronchi; the left bronchus and the right bronchus. The bronchi are branches of the trachea that supply the left and right lungs.

The right bronchus is wider and more vertical than the left. Both are further divided into a network of narrower passages called bronchioles.

Bronchioles

As mentioned above, bronchioles are narrow passageways which branch from the bronchi. They can branch many times and end in tiny air sacs called alveoli.

Alveoli

Alveoli are extremely tiny, thin-walled, elastic air sacs. They are lined by a flat epithelium and surrounded by pulmonary capillaries. The barrier between the gas in the alveoli and the blood in the vessels is so thin that oxygen and carbon dioxide can pass across it.

Lungs

The lungs are a pair of conical organs each surrounded by a specialised membrane called the *pleura*. The pleura consists of two layers moistened by a special fluid, resembling lymph, which acts as a lubricant enabling the two surfaces to glide smoothly over each other during respiration.

Intercostal muscles

There are both external and internal intercostal muscles. Both sets lie between the ribs. They are responsible for raising and lowering the chest during *inspiration* (breathing in) and *expiration* (breathing out).

Diaphragm

The diaphragm is a sheet of muscle that separates the thorax from the abdomen. It is a little unusual in that when it is contracted it becomes flattened and when relaxed it is dome-shaped. The muscle originates from the tip of the sternum, the lower ribs and the cartilages of the lumbar vertebrae and is inserted into the central aponeurosis (a flattened-out tendon). Three openings in the diaphragm allow for the passage of the oesophagus, the aorta and the vena cava. The flattening of the diaphragm increases the volume of the chest cavity, aiding inspiration. Relaxing the diaphragm decreases the volume of the chest cavity, aiding expiration.

How the respiratory system works

The processes of respiration can be summarised in four parts:

* Movement of air in and out of the lungs.
* Free passage of air down the airways.
* Gaseous exchange.
* Control of respiration.

Movement of air in and out of the lungs

During inspiration the intercostal muscles contract, moving the rib-cage upwards and outwards, and the diaphragm contracts downwards to a more flattened position. This causes the thorax to increase in volume, hence decreasing the pressure in the chest cavity. This causes a pressure difference to develop between the inside and outside of the lungs. Air moves from the region of higher pressure (outside the lungs) to the region of lower pressure (inside the lungs) until the pressure difference is removed.

During expiration the diaphragm and intercostal muscles relax and the ribcage returns to the normal position. This has the effect of reducing the volume within the thorax, increasing the air pressure in the lungs, forcing air out of the lungs.

Free passage of air down the airways

As air is breathed in through the nose it passes over hairs and mucous which filter and warm the air. The air passes through the naso-pharynx where it is further filtered and warmed, to the larynx and down the trachea. The trachea also contains mucous secreting ciliated cells which remove any debris from the inhaled air not already dealt with. The air then moves into the bronchial tree, through the bronchi and bronchioles to reach the alveoli.

The air retraces this journey during expiration.

Gaseous exchange

In the lungs, oxygen from the inspired air in the alveolus passes across the alveolar membrane and the capillary walls to combine with haemoglobin in the red blood cells. Simultaneously, carbon dioxide diffuses back from the blood into the alveolar air so that it can be exhaled.

Control of Respiration

Control of respiration is achieved through both chemical and neurological means. Respiration is controlled by nerve cells in the medulla oblongata in what is known as the *respiratory centre*. It is further controlled by chemoreceptors in the walls of the aorta and carotid arteries which are sensitive to changes in oxygen and carbon dioxide concentrations in the blood.

USEFUL INFORMATION

Air is composed of approximately:
* *Nitrogen, 78%.*
* *Oxygen, 21%.*
* *Inert gases, 0.07%.*
* *Carbon dioxide, 0.03% (variable).*
* *Water vapour (variable).*

PROGRESS CHECK

1 State the composition of air.
2 Describe briefly the mechanism of breathing.

The digestive system

The digestive system is concerned with the taking in and breakdown of food. There are two phases to digestion, mechanical and chemical.

The digestive system consists of the alimentary tract or canal and the glands secreting digestive juices which act upon the food matter.

The alimentary canal is a passage over 9 meters long leading from the mouth to the rectum. It is lined throughout with a mucous membrane which lubricates the system. Muscular walls act upon the foodstuffs

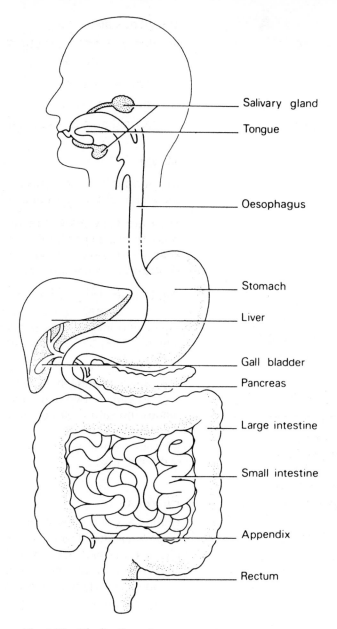

Salivary gland

Tongue

Oesophagus

Stomach

Liver

Gall bladder

Pancreas

Large intestine

Small intestine

Appendix

Rectum

Fig. 1.22 *The digestive system*

eaten and help their passage along the alimentary canal. The alimentary canal consists of:

* Mouth.
* Pharynx.
* Oesophagus.
* Stomach.
* Small intestine.
* Large intestine.

39

The glands are:

- Salivary glands – secreting saliva in the mouth.
- Gastric glands – secreting gastric juices in the stomach.
- Pancreas – secreting pancreatic juice in the duodenum.
- Liver – secreting bile in the duodenum.
- Intestinal glands – secreting intestinal juice in the small intestine.

Mouth

Digestion commences mechanically and chemically in the mouth with the action of the teeth and salivary glands respectively.

There are 32 permanent teeth in the adult mouth of four types. Each type of tooth has a specific function in the breakdown of food; the *incisors* are adapted to break off food, the *canines* are adapted to tear at meat and the *premolars* and *molars* are adapted to grind and chew.

The tongue also plays a part in mechanical digestion. It consists of striated voluntary muscle attached mainly to the mandible and hyoid bones and helps in the swallowing action by forming the food into a suitably sized ball, or *bolus*, and moving it to the pharynx at the back of the mouth.

The salivary glands in the mouth begin chemical digestion. There are two parotid glands, two mandibular glands and two sublingual glands (the names indicate their positions in the mouth). They secrete a watery substance called *saliva* which contains the digestive enzyme *ptyalin* (amylase) which is involved in the first stage of the digestion of carbohydrates.

Pharynx

At the back of the mouth lies the pharynx which is about 13 cm long and leads backwards from the mouth. It consists of three areas – the naso pharynx, the oral pharynx and the larygeal pharynx. The oral pharynx is shared by both air and food and the larygeal pharynx merges with the oesophagus. When food is swallowed, the pharynx contracts forcing food downwards into the oesophagus.

Oesophagus

The oesophagus is a muscular tube 25–30 cm long leading from the pharynx to the stomach. It is composed of voluntary and involuntary muscle fibres which work in a wave-like motion called *peristalsis* to propel food into the stomach.

Stomach

The stomach is a muscular sac-like organ placed on the left side of the abdominal cavity beneath the diaphragm. At either end of the stomach are valves, called *sphincters*, which allow or restrict the movement of food into or out of the stomach. The *cardiac sphincter* lies between the oesophagus and the top of the stomach and the *pyloric sphincter* lies between the bottom of the stomach and the duodenum.

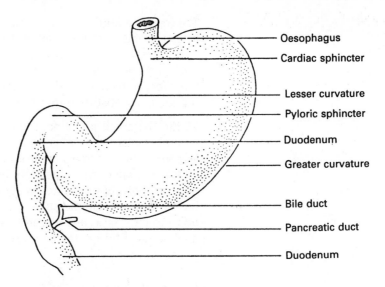

Oesophagus
Cardiac sphincter
Lesser curvature
Pyloric sphincter
Duodenum
Greater curvature
Bile duct
Pancreatic duct
Duodenum

Fig. 1.23 *The stomach*

The stomach has several distinct layers. The outermost layer is called the *peritoneum* and its main function is to prevent friction with other organs in the abdominal cavity. The peritoneum is a serous membrane, that is it produces a fluid called serum which acts as a lubricant. Next there is a muscular layer, then a layer which is composed of connective tissue and is rich in blood vessels. Forming the stomach lining is a mucous layer. The layers of the stomach have the ability to expand and contract according to the amount of food consumed. The surface of the inner stomach is convoluted. This provides a greater surface area for the action of secreted acidic gastric juices on the food. Food is held in the stomach until it becomes liquefied and has been partially digested.

Chemical digestion continues in the stomach. Protein digestion commences; proteins are broken down to *peptones*. Gastric juice contains *hydrochloric acid* and the enzymes *pepsin* and *rennin*. The acid is antiseptic in action and provides the correct medium for the digestive juices to work in.

Mechanical digestion is also continued in the stomach. The food is churned with strong muscular movements and leaves the stomach in a series of gushes.

Some substances ingested are absorbed directly into the body from the stomach; these include water, alcohol and glucose.

Small intestine

This part of the digestive tract leads from the stomach to the large intestine and is 6–7.4 metres in length. It has three main sections; the *duodenum*, the *jejunum* and the *ileum*.

The duodenum is the first part of the small intestine and is attached to the back of the abdominal wall by peritoneum. It is approximately 24 cm long and curves like the letter C. Lying within the curve is the pancreas.

The jejunum and ileum form most of the total length of the small intestine and lie to the front of the abdominal cavity. The structure of the small intestine is similar to the stomach externally but internally it is puckered and covered with hair-like projections called *villi*. These have the effect of increasing the surface area of the small intestine. Digestion products are absorbed into the villi.

Within the small intestine, the digestion of protein, carbohydrate and fats takes place. Enzymes from three types of digestive juice – *pancreatic juice* from the pancreas, *bile* from the liver, *succus entericus* from the small intestine – affect this digestion. Peptones from the stomach are broken down to polypeptides and finally to amino-acids; carbohydrates are broken down to simple sugars, e.g. glucose; fats and oils are broken down to fatty acids and glycerol. Fatty acids and glycerol after absorption may be used for energy by muscles in activity, or stored.

Large intestine

The large intestine is the last stage of the alimentary tract and begins at the ileum and ends at the rectum. It is about 1.5 metres in length and is divided into three parts:

- the ascending colon
- the transverse colon
- the descending colon.

The first part of the ascending colon consists of a lined pouch called the *caecum* from which extends the *vermiform appendix*. It contains the *ileo-caecal valve* which allows on-flow, but prevents back-flow, of intestinal contents. The remainder of food undigested, plus roughage and unabsorbed digestive juice pass from the small intestine into the large intestine in a liquid form. Here the water is reabsorbed and the solid faeces are formed.

Glands of the digestive system

The liver

The liver is the largest gland in the body, weighing between 1 and 2.3 kg. It is situated in the upper part of the abdominal cavity and consists of four lobes. Blood rich in nutrients is supplied to the liver via the *hepatic portal vein* which carries blood from the stomach, spleen, pancreas and the intestines. Arterial blood is supplied to the liver via the *hepatic artery*. The right and left *hepatic ducts* carry bile from the liver to the gall bladder. The main digestive functions of the liver are:

- Production of bile, which together with lipase from the pancreas commences the first stage of fat digestion.
- Synthesis of vitamin A from carotene.
- Storage of vitamins, namely B12, A, D, E, K and iron.

The pancreas

The pancreas is a pale grey gland weighing approximately 60 g. It is situated high on the left side of the abdominal cavity behind the stomach. The pancreas consists of a large number of lobules made up of

USEFUL INFORMATION

The pancreas is both an endocrine and an exocrine gland as it secretes hormones (see p. 34) and also has a digestive function.

42

small alveoli and these secrete pancreatic juice which contains the enzymes *lipase, trypsin, chymotrypsin* and *amylase*. Lipase converts fats into monoglycerides, diglycerides and fatty acids. Trypsin and chymotrypsin convert peptones (protein) into polypeptides. Amylase converts carbohydrates (starch) into maltose.

| PROGRESS CHECK | 1 Explain briefly the digestive process. |
| | 2 What are the main functions of the liver. |

The urinary system

The urinary system consists of:
* The kidneys.
* Ureters.
* Bladder.
* Urethra.

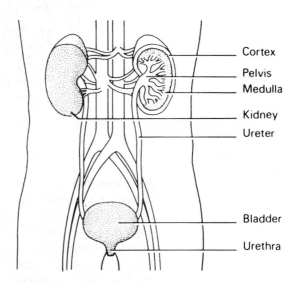

Fig. 1.24 *The urinary system*

The kidneys

There are two kidneys, each approximately 11 cm in length by 6 cm in width. They lie high on the posterior wall of the abdomen. Each kidney consists of an outer layer called a fibrous capsule, a *cortex*, an inner *medulla* which contains *renal pyramids* and the pelvis.

Each kidney receives blood at very high pressure through a renal artery. Once inside the kidney, the artery divides into smaller capillaries which carry the blood to tiny cup-shaped structures called *glomerular capsules*. The glomerular capsule is the beginning of a length of narrow tube, approximately 3 cm long called a *nephron*. Urine is produced in the nephrons.

Formation of urine

The capillary inside each glomerular capsule divides into a tiny bundle of inter-twined blood vessels called a *glomerulus*. Blood pressure is so high in this area that liquid is forced out through the capillary walls into the space inside the glomerular capsule. This liquid is known as *glomerular filtrate*. It contains urea to be excreted together with many useful substances (e.g. glucose, amino acids, mineral salts, vitamins and large amounts of water) which the body cannot afford to lose. These substances are reabsorbed in the nephron.

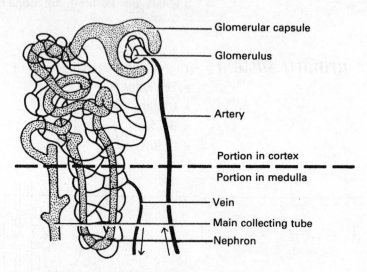

Fig. 1.25 *Internal structure of a kidney*

Reabsorption

Glomerular filtrate flows out of the glomerular capsules into the tubular part of each nephron; it is here that reabsorption occurs. The walls of the nephron extract useful substances from the filtrate and these pass into blood flowing through capillaries surrounding the nephron. What is left now is *urine*, which consists of waste products such as urea, uric acid and small amounts of mineral salts.

The ureters, bladder and urethra

A thin tube called a *ureter* which is attached to the concave side of each kidney conveys the urine to a single large bag called the *bladder*. The bladder has only one exit, a tube called the *urethra*, which leads to the body's surface. The bladder end of the urethra is closed by means of a sphincter. Urine drains continuously out of the kidneys into the ureters, where it is forced downwards into the bladder by wave-like contractions. The bladder stretches and expands as it fills with urine. When the bladder is full, the stretching stimulates sensory nerve endings in its walls which convey nerve impulses to the brain letting you know when your bladder must be emptied. The sphincter muscles around the urethra are then voluntarily relaxed allowing urine to drain from the bladder through the urethra and out of the body.

PROGRESS CHECK

1 Explain briefly how urine is produced.

2 Describe the appearance of a kidney.

Anatomy of the female breast

The breasts are the accessory glands of the female reproductive system and are composed of fatty, fibrous and glandular tissues. Breasts mature in the female at puberty under the influence of the female hormones oestrogen and progesterone.

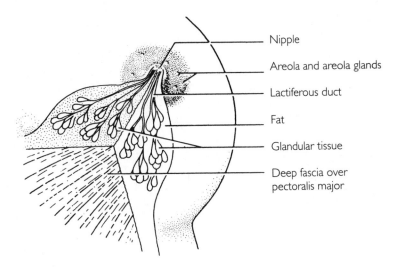

Nipple

Areola and areola glands

Lactiferous duct

Fat

Glandular tissue

Deep fascia over pectoralis major

Fig. 1.26 *Section through the breast*

The breasts are structured for breast feeding with each consisting of about 15–20 lobes of glandular tissue. These are formed from lobules and are connected by areolar tissue, blood vessels and ducts. Each lobule is made up from tiny little sacs called alveoli which collectively form lactiferous ducts. These converge towards the nipple (or *areolar*) where they form a *lactiferous sinus* whose function is to act as reservoir for milk in the event of lactation.

Fatty tissue covers the entire surface of the breast whilst fibrous tissue, in conjunction with the pectoral muscle group lying directly underneath on the chest wall, provides support for the breast.

POINT TO NOTE ▷ *Suspensory ligaments in the form of fibrous tissue give the breasts their firm contour. The firm contour decreases as we age. It is therefore extremely important to wear a good, properly fitted, supporting bra at all times.*

PROGRESS CHECK

1 What is the main function of the female breast.

2 Explain the importance of the pectoratis muscle group.

KEY TERMS

You need to know what these words and phrases mean. Go back through the chapter to find out.

Cells and tissues
Epidermis
Dermis
Subcutis
The skeletal system
Types of muscular tissue
The heart

Blood and lymphatic circulation
The neurological system
Endocrine glands
The respiratory system
The digestive system
The kidneys
The female breast

---

2 Advice on dietary control and exercise

After working through this chapter you will be able to:

➤ list the different nutrients required for a balanced diet
➤ identify the different food sources for the different nutrients
➤ list the reasons why people may wish to gain or lose weight
➤ list different types of diet
➤ recognise the different body types
➤ identify a number of postural problems
➤ list the components of fitness
➤ understand the factors that should be considered when offering corrective exercise home care advice.

As many clients attend health spas and clinics to support them in a weight loss programme, it is important that the therapist has an understanding of basic nutrition. It must however be stressed that the role of the therapist is not that of a dietician who undertakes specialist training in this field. Health spas employ medical staff to carry out a client's initial consultation and will refer them to the dietitian if a special diet is needed due to medical conditions such as diabetes or if the client wishes to lose weight. Many therapists in salons work in close liaison with doctors, particularly if offering specialised treatments such as alpha hydroxy acids or collagen injections, and some salons extend their range of treatments to include dietary advice under medical supervision. It is strongly recommended that the therapist should only supplement their clients' weight loss programmes with information on healthy eating. The therapist must refer the client to their doctor if they have any underlying medical problems or a serious weight condition.

Basic nutrition

In order for our body to operate efficiently it requires a well-balanced diet. In general a normal varied diet will provide all the nutrients required for health, though during illness or pregnancy the diet will require additional supplements, e.g. iron is often needed to supplement the diet of expectant mothers. During the latter half of this century there has been a greater tendency for mothers to take up employment and this trend, along with the advancements in convenience foods, has been responsible for a move away from the traditional diet. However, more recently, people have become health conscious and realise that trends in lifestyle may lead to an unbalanced diet. Many people now pay more care and attention to their diet.

47

Nutrition, in conjunction with digestion, is the process by which the body absorbs foodstuffs and converts them to substances that it requires for life. Food is made up of differing amounts of substances and these can either be used directly by our bodies or converted into other substances our bodies need. The types of food required by an healthy individual are; proteins, carbohydrates, fats, water, roughage, mineral elements and vitamins.

Proteins

Proteins are used by the body for the growth and repair of body tissues. They also act as a secondary source of energy. Proteins are broken down during digestion into amino acids. Proteins are made up of varying amounts of different amino acids and can be sub-divided into two categories; first class proteins and second class proteins.

First class proteins

First class proteins are those that contain all the essential amino acids required by the body. Sources of first class proteins are meat, milk, eggs, fish and soya beans.

Second class proteins

Second class proteins are those that do not contain all the essential amino acids. Sources of second class proteins are pulses and nuts.

POINTS TO NOTE ▷

● Proteins are made up of carbon, hydrogen, oxygen and nitrogen. Some also contain phosphorous and sulphur.

● Most sources of first class protein are of animal origin. Vegetarian diets, particularly vegan diets, can be deficient in certain essential amino acids.

Carbohydrates

Carbohydrates provide the body with energy. If an excess of carbohydrates is eaten the body coverts them and stores them as fat. Sources of carbohydrates are starchy and sugary foods such as cereals, bread, potatoes, sugar, vegetables and fruits.

Carbohydrates are digested in the alimentary canal and are absorbed into the body in the form of monosaccharides, the simplest chemical form in which carbohydrates can exist. Examples of monosaccharides are glucose, fructose and galactose.

POINTS TO NOTE ▷

● Carbohydrates are made up of carbon, hydrogen and oxygen.

● Starch forms the larger proportion of the carbohydrates we eat in our food. It must be broken down by the body into simple sugars before it can be used as an energy source.

● The body breaks down complex sugars and starch into glucose which is the form in which fuel is transported around to the different organs of the body.

Fats

The body needs a certain quantity of fat to protect organs, provide insulation, transport fat-soluble vitamins and provide energy. Excess fat in the diet is converted into fatty acids and stored until it is needed. Fats come from either animal or vegetable sources.

Examples of foods containing animal fats are meat, cheese, butter, milk and eggs. Vegetable oils and margarine contain vegetable fats.

Cholesterol is a fat-like substance which is produced naturally in the bodies of all animals. A high level of cholesterol in the blood encourages the build up of deposits of fat on the inside walls of arteries which can lead to heart problems.

USEFUL INFORMATION

Approximately two thirds of the body weight is made up of water.

POINTS TO NOTE ▷

* *Fats are made up of carbon, hydrogen and oxygen, though in different proportions to carbohydrates.*
* *Animal fats are known to increase the cholesterol level in the body.*
* *Fats have double the energy value of carbohydrates.*
* *Fats are slow to digest and produce linoleic acid which is needed for healthy skin.*

USEFUL INFORMATION

* *When each carbon atom in a fat molecule has the maximum number of hydrogen atoms attached to it, the fat is known as a saturated fat.*
* *Differing patterns of carbon and hydrogen atoms produce mono-unsaturated and polyunsaturated fats.*
* *Vegetable fats kept at room temperature tend to be liquid or soft, whereas animal fats tend to be hard.*
* *Fats contain only small quantities of water.*

Water

A large proportion of the body weight is made up of water. Water is found in the blood and tissue fluids and aids in digestion, maintaining the body temperature and health of cells. It also dilutes waste products and assists in their elimination. It is found throughout the body in varying quantities and is essential to life. The body excretes around two litres of water per day in the form of urine and perspiration. The body re-balances its fluid loss by absorbing water from drinks and food. The majority of foods we eat contain some water.

Roughage

Roughage is a nutrient that is not digestible but is required by the body to assist in the digestion process, in particular excretion. It provides the diet with bulk, helping to satisfy the appetite and provides a medium on which peristalsis can work, hence aiding the movement of food through the alimentary canal.

POINT TO NOTE ▷ *Roughage is sometimes referred to as fibre.*

Mineral elements

Minerals are needed by the body to maintain health. They are not required in large quantities in the diet.

Calcium

Calcium is needed for the formation and maintenance of healthy teeth and bones and for muscular activity. It can be found in foods such as milk, cheese and eggs.

Iodine

Iodine is essential for the formation of the hormone thyroxine from the thyroid gland. It is only needed in very small quantities and can be found in foods such as watercress, seafood and iodised salt.

Iron

Iron is used by the body to manufacture haemoglobin. Women generally require more iron in their diet than men as they lose blood, and therefore iron, during menstruation. During pregnancy expectant mothers often need to supplement their diet with additional iron to maintain their own health and that of the foetus. Iron can be found in foods such as liver and green vegetables, e.g. spinach.

Magnesium

Magnesium is needed by the body for metabolism and the composition of bones, nerves and muscles. It can be found in foods such as green vegetables, wholegrain cereals and lentils.

Manganese

Manganese is necessary for metabolism and can be found in foods such as kidneys, lentils, almonds, apricots, wheatgerm and watercress.

Phosphorus

Phosphorus is needed for the formation of teeth and bones. It is a constituent of cells and plays a part in the maintenance of body fluid balance and aids in the utilisation of energy from foods. It can be found in foods such as cheese, eggs, meat, fish, yeast, wheatgerm and green vegetables.

Potassium

Potassium is needed to maintain the body's fluid balance and is also involved in the functioning of nerves and muscles. It can be found in the majority of foods, especially milk, cheese, seafood, bananas, spinach, butter and baked potatoes.

Sodium

Sodium is required to maintain the fluid balance of the body. It also plays an important role in the transmission of impulses from the nerves and in muscular contraction. It can be found in the majority of foods, in particular salt.

Sulphur

Sulphur helps with the formation of body tissues and can be found in foods such as eggs, fish, cheese, meat and beans.

USEFUL INFORMATION

Some vegan diets can be deficient in zinc.

Trace elements

Trace elements are found in extremely small quantities within the body and are needed for a variety of body processes such as digestion. Examples of trace elements are copper, cobalt, fluorine and zinc. Zinc is found in foods such as fish and nuts and is important for a healthy skin.

POINTS TO NOTE ▷

* *Mineral elements are often called mineral salts.*
* *Deficiency in iron leads to anaemia.*
* *Calcium absorption diminishes in females over 50.*

Vitamins

Vitamins have no energy value but are essential organic substances required in small quantities for health and certain chemical activities of the body.

They can be categorised into two groups:

* Water-soluble vitamins such as B complex and C.
* Fat-soluble vitamins such as A, D, E and K.

USEFUL INFORMATION

The liver can convert carotene, which is found in foods such as carrots and spinach, into vitamin A.

Vitamin A (retinol)

Vitamin A is needed for the growth of the majority of body cells and is particularly important for healthy eyesight. Deficiency in vitamin A can lead to poor night vision and dry skin. Good sources of vitamin A are milk, butter, cream, eggs, cheese, carrots, green vegetables and oily fish, e.g. sardines.

Vitamin B complex

Vitamin B includes a complex of vitamins:

* Vitamin B1 (thiamine) helps the nervous system to function and controls the release of energy from carbohydrates. Examples of food sources are wheatgerm, offal, yeast, eggs and nuts.
* Vitamin B2 (riboflavin) is needed for energy and health of the mouth and skin. It can be found in foods such as eggs, cheese, kidneys and liver. It is resistant to heat but can be destroyed by sunlight.
* Pantothenic acid is essential for the body's nervous system and in the burning of fat for energy. Examples of food containing pantothenic acid are liver, egg yolk and vegetables. It is present in most types of food.
* Vitamin B6 (pyridoxine) helps with many of the body's functions and is obtained from foods such as brewer's yeast, bread, wholegrain cereal, milk, eggs and liver.
* Niacin or nicotinic acid is crucial for the utilisation of energy and healthy skin. It plays parts in both the digestive and nervous systems. It can be found in food such as liver, eggs, cheese, brewer's yeast and bread.

● Folic acid is important for the formation of red blood cells and can be found in foods such as liver, kidneys and fresh green vegetables.

● Vitamin B12 is needed in the body for the production of red blood cells. Examples of food sources are meat and dairy products.

● Biotin is required for healthy skin and hair. It is produced naturally by the body and can be obtained from such food stuffs as liver, yeast, kidneys and egg yolk.

Vitamin C (ascorbic acid)

Vitamin C assists in the formation of connective tissue, the absorption of iron and the development and maintenance of healthy bones. It can be found in foods such as vegetables and citrus fruits, e.g. oranges

---

POINT TO NOTE ▷ *Some vitamins such as B and C are sensitive to heat and can be destroyed in the cooking process.*

Vitamin D (calciferol)

Vitamin D assists in depositing phosphorous and calcium in the bones and is therefore required for the formation of healthy, strong bones and teeth. Examples of foods with a rich supply of vitamin D are cheese, eggs, margarine, butter and fatty fish. The body can produce vitamin D when exposed to sunlight and is able to store it in the liver.

Vitamin E (tocopherol)

The function of vitamin E is not known, however it is thought that a deficiency prevents growth. It can be found in foods such as peanuts, milk, vegetable oils, eggs, fish, wholemeal bread and cereals. Deep-frying destroys a lot of this vitamin.

Vitamin K

Vitamin K is needed for the clotting mechanism of blood. It can be obtained from green vegetables, fruit and liver.

ACTIVITY

Compile lists of a child's and an adult's daily food intake and note the different nutrients that will have been absorbed by their bodies.

PROGRESS CHECK

1 List the nutrients required for a balanced diet.

2 Give an example of a good food source for each of the following nutrients:
   a protein   c fats   e iron and calcium.
   b carbohydrate   d vitamins A and C

3 State how each of the following is used by the body:
   a protein   d calcium   g vitamin C
   b carbohydrate   e iron   h vitamin D.
   c fats   f vitamin A

Metabolism

Metabolism is the process by which the body makes use of the food it takes in and utilises it for energy, growth and general health. The body metabolises basic food elements in two general ways:

* Catabolism is the way in which the body releases energy by breaking down food.
* Anabolism is the way in which the body builds up or utilises cell structures from digested food materials.

Calorific requirements

The body needs a well-balanced diet to meet its individual daily requirements. The calorific requirement of an individual is the amount of energy the body needs to stay warm and do any work required of it. Fats have a higher calorific value than carbohydrates, i.e. they contains more energy per unit weight, and carbohydrates have a higher calorific value than proteins. As people vary in size, age, gender and way of life, each individual will have different nutritional needs. It is therefore impossible to state a general energy requirement to suit everybody. Women generally require less energy than men; manual workers require more energy than sedentary office workers; older people require less energy than younger people.

Basal metabolism

The basal metabolism is the minimum energy output required by the body for vital functioning, e.g. respiration, heart beat, peristalsis, etc. The basal metabolic rate varies according to gender, age, life style and body size. It also tends to decrease with age. If the body absorbs more energy from foods than it needs for basal metabolism and the work it does (e.g. exercise), it will store the excess as fat around the body.

POINTS TO NOTE ▷

* *As the body ages the basal metabolic rate will fall by an average of 5% every 10 years.*
* *Regular exercise increases the metabolic rate as muscle cells burn up more calories than fat cells even when at rest.*

Diets

Social and peer-group pressures regarding the way individuals look can create a great deal of stress in people's lives. One of the major influencing factors in how people feel about themselves often relates to how they truly feel about their body shape and size. It cannot be stated that obese people are more unhappy with their appearance than extremely thin people as feelings are individual and other factors in people's lives often alter their emotions, e.g. the excitement of a new job or home, or a loving relationship can all detract from past insecurities and can bring about weight loss or gain! There are a variety of reasons why a person may be over or under weight, e.g. a lack of, or excessive exercise, poor diet. Some people suffer with weight problems due to medical conditions such as an over or under active thyroid gland.

A general indicator to assess a client's frame size is the circumference of their wrist:

- *14 cm (5 $\frac{1}{2}$ inches) = Small*
- *15.25 cm (6 inches) = Medium*
- *16.5 cm (6 $\frac{1}{2}$ inches) = Large*

For figure assessment, when measuring a client:

- *Remember to consider their modesty – only expose the areas you need to measure.*
- *Do not pull the tape measure tight.*
- *Always record the measurements accurately.*

There are a variety of reasons why people may wish to loose or gain weight including:

- To feel healthy and fit.
- To feel happy with their appearance.
- To restore their figure after childbirth.
- To prevent coronary conditions.

It is a common misconception that it is only women who worry about weight problems. In today's society men take a lot more time and effort over their appearance and although some may not show it they often suffer in the same way as women if they are not happy with the way they look. People may wish to diet to improve their total shape whilst others may feel that they have problems with particular areas such as the abdomen, thighs and hips. For whatever reason a person wishes to loose or gain weight they must be sensible in adjusting their diet to ensure it meets the body's nutritional requirements and suits their lifestyle.

There are many books available on different types of diet and fact sheets available through doctors, hospitals and slimming organisations. The important thing to remember if wishing to loose weight is that the body stores excess energy obtained from fats, carbohydrates and proteins in the form of fat around the body. As a person continually takes in surplus energy requirements, the fat cells will increase in size and thus they will gain more and more weight. Therefore the diet will need to be balanced and they will need to increase their energy output to burn up the excess fat. For those wishing to gain weight it is often quite difficult to increase the intake of foods with a high calorific value and the process of weight gain for many people is a slow and arduous task.

POINTS TO NOTE ▷
- *Weight loss should be slow and controlled, as often people who lose weight rapidly find it returns fairly quickly.*
- *Individuals develop different eating habits, e.g. some people like to nibble whilst others like full meals and others need to satisfy a sweet tooth.*

Women

ft ins	cm	Small lbs	kgs	Medium lbs	kgs	Large lbs	kgs
4 10	147	102–111	46–50	109–121	49–55	118–131	54–59
4 11	150	103–113	47–51	111–123	50–56	120–134	55–61
5 0	152	104–115	47–52	113–126	51–57	122–137	56–62
5 1	155	106–118	48–54	115–129	52–59	125–140	57–61
5 2	158	108–121	49–55	118–132	54–60	128–143	58–65
5 3	160	111–124	50–56	121–135	55–61	131–147	59–67
5 4	163	114–127	52–58	124–138	56–63	134–151	61–69
5 5	165	117–130	53–59	127–141	58–64	137–155	62–70
5 6	168	120–133	55–60	130–144	59–65	140–159	63–72
5 7	170	123–136	56–62	133–147	60–67	143–163	65–74
5 8	173	126–139	57–63	136–150	62–68	146–167	66–76
5 9	175	129–142	59–64	139–153	63–69	149–170	68–77
5 10	178	132–145	60–66	142–156	64–71	152–173	69–79
5 11	180	135–148	61–67	145–159	66–72	155–176	70–80
6 0	183	138–151	63–69	148–162	67–74	158–179	72–81

Men

ft ins	cm	Small lbs	Medium lbs	Large lbs
5 2	158	128–134	131–141	138–150
5 3	160	130–136	133–144	140–153
5 4	163	132–138	135–145	142–156
5 5	165	134–140	137–148	144–160
5 6	168	136–142	139–151	146–164
5 7	170	138–145	142–154	149–168
5 8	173	140–148	145–157	152–172
5 9	175	142–151	148–160	155–176
5 10	178	144–154	151–163	158–180
5 11	180	146–157	154–166	161–184
6 0	183	149–160	157–170	164–188
6 1	185	152–164	160–174	168–192
6 2	188	155–168	164–178	172–197
6 3	190	158–172	167–182	176–202
6 4	193	162–176	171–187	181–207

Fig. 2.1 *Charts to show an example of accepted weight norms of gender, height and frame size*

Types of diet

There are many types of diet available to suit individual requirements. Some of these are outlined below.

Calorie controlled diet

This type of diet limits the quantity of calories the individual takes in per day, but enables them to select the types of food they eat. It is also a useful diet for those who eat out socially as it allows them to save calories for that special meal without everyone they eat with focusing on the fact that they are on a diet. It can also assist those who have a sweet tooth by enabling them to save calories for a treat.

High protein diet

A high protein diet is suitable for people who want to build muscles. However, a diet high in protein can still produce excess energy requirements as protein is a secondary source of energy. Also, protein type foods often contain saturated fats which can increase the body's cholesterol level.

Low fat diet

A low fat diet will obviously reduce the main energy source from outside the body. Some of the fat which was laid down and stored when the body was consuming an excess to the body's requirements is utilised instead.

Low carbohydrate diet

A low carbohydrate diet means reducing the quantity of sugars and starch in the diet. Some people find this hard to do particularly if they have a sweet tooth. As the body obtains most of its daily energy requirement from carbohydrates, it works by reducing the readily available energy. The body calls on its reserve of energy, the stock-pile of fat!

High fibre diet

A high fibre diet provides a lot of bulk to the diet which generally makes the dieter feel full. High fibre diets also improve bowel conditions such as constipation.

Vegetarian diets

Over the years many people have opted to become vegetarians. There are two types of vegetarian:

- Lacto-vegetarians, who do eat some animal products such as milk, cheese and eggs.
- Vegans, who do not eat any form of animal produce.

Health diets

Health diets are prescribed by doctors or nutritionists for the benefit of their patients' health. Examples of people who require health diets are coronary sufferers and diabetics.

Commercial diet products

There are a large variety of products which can be purchased over the counter in many shops. They include solid food substances, e.g. diet bars, and powders which are mixed with water to produce liquid meals. The main problem with commercial diet products is that people tend to totally replace their diet with them and do not balance their diet nutritionally. Often these products' calorific values are way below the body's daily needs.

Slimming clubs

Over recent years the number of slimming and similar clubs has increased rapidly. Many people gain support and comfort from other dieters.

POINT TO NOTE ▷ *It is important with all diets to ensure that the body receives balanced nutrients to maintain health, repair and growth.*

ACTIVITY	Analyse the dietary habits of two colleagues and research their daily calorific intake.

Alternative weight control

There are a variety of alternative ways in which weight can be controlled:

- Acupuncture. This can prove to be quite a costly method depending how quickly the dieter responds to treatment, however many people find it helps suppress their appetite.
- Hypnosis. Depending upon an individual's response to hypnotherapy this method may encourage weight loss.
- Cosmetic surgery. This is a fairly drastic and expensive method to remove surplus fat.
- Tablets. There are a variety of slimming tablets that can be purchased over the counter. These are taken a number of hours before eating to suppress the appetite.
- Drugs. Doctors sometimes prescribe drugs to people whose life is threatened by their weight to help suppress their appetite.

ACTIVITY	Research the alternative weight loss methods available in your local area, noting the cost and duration of treatments.

Eating problems

There are a variety of different types of eating problems, some of which can prove to be fatal.

Stress-induced eating

Stress affects everyone differently, but it can be noted that weight is either lost or gained according to how it effects an individual's eating patterns. Some people eat more under stress as they often take comfort from eating, whilst others eat a great deal less as they find their appetite reduced. Quite often when the anxieties disappear the normal eating pattern will gradually re-emerge. It is important to note that help in some form should be sought to cope with the problem creating the stress, particularly if rapid weight loss is noted. There are many self-help groups for people suffering with stress depending on the cause, e.g. living with cancer, loosing a child. However it may be just the support of family or friends that is needed to reduce anxiety and bring comfort or a relaxing massage.

57

Bulimia nervosa

Bulimia nervosa is a disease where sufferers will 'binge' and afterwards make themselves sick. It is sometimes very difficult to realise that a person close to you is suffering with this disease, particularly in the early stages as they mainly eat in front of people. It is important that medical help is sought as soon as possible.

Anorexia nervosa

Anorexia nervosa is a slimmer's disease where sufferers slowly starve themselves of food. This disease is often brought on by social pressure to be slim. The sufferer starts by dieting, quite often drastically, to loose weight. Once the weight is lost the suffer still perceives him/herself as 'too fat' and comes to believe that any food he/she eats will increase his/her weight. This can be a life-threatening disease and medical help should be sought as soon as possible.

Figure and postural analysis

In order to perform an effective body-treatment consultation the therapist must have an understanding of the figure and postural problems that a client may have.

Body types

Body types are generally categorised into three types; *ectomorph*, *mesomorph* and *endomorph*. However it should be noted that the majority of people tend to be a combination of the categorised body types.

The ectomorph

Ectomorphs tend to be recognised by:

* Narrow shoulders and hips.
* Long bones.
* Not much muscle bulk.
* Low percentage of fat.
* General lack of curves.

The mesomorph

Mesomorphs tend to be recognised by:

* Athletic build.
* Well-developed shoulders.
* Slim, 'boyish' hips.
* Well-toned muscles.
* Low percentage of fat.

The endomorph

Endomorphs tend to be recognised by:

* Rounded shoulders.
* Heavy build.
* Higher percentage of fat to muscle bulk.
* Inclination to be overweight.

USEFUL INFORMATION

Although the appearance of the body can be altered through diet and exercise the actual body type remains constant through life.

Fig. 2.2 *Ectomorph*   **Fig. 2.3** *Mesomorph*   **Fig. 2.4** *Endomorph*

Good posture

It is rare to find perfect posture. This is mainly due to the lifestyles that we lead: company representatives who spend a great deal of their day driving often suffer with tense, round shoulders; busy mothers who carry young children around on their hips or carry heavy shopping bags on one side whilst holding their child's hand for example often suffer with scoliosis.

We naturally take notice of the person who holds him/herself well. A person with good posture often creates a good first impression compared to the person who slouches. Watch men and women when they are attracted by a member of the opposite sex they automatically react by stretching their bodies upright! Besides enhancing the body's appearance good posture also maximises the lung capacity which obviously has a beneficial effect on the body.

Points to look for in good posture
1 The head should not abnormally extend or retract beyond the mid line.
2 The arms, when relaxed, should lie evenly.
3 The spinal column should be straight.
4 The distances from the right and left scapulae to the spine should be even.
5 The abdomen should appear flat.
6 The waist curves should be level.
7 The buttocks should not protrude abnormally.
8 The legs and knees should be straight and facing forwards.

Fig. 2.5 *Correct postural stance (lateral view)*

9 The feet should face forwards and should be either together or slightly apart.

10 The body weight should be evenly distributed.

If an imaginary, lateral line is drawn down the side of the body it should pass in a straight line through the ear, shoulder, elbow, waist, hip, knee and ankle. Trainee therapists often use a plumbline to assist in postural analysis.

PROGRESS CHECK

1 State four reasons why clients may wish to gain or lose weight.

2 Explain briefly four different types of diet.

3 Describe three different eating problems.

4 Name the three main body types and for each give a brief description of how you would recognise them.

5 What points would you look for to establish good posture in a client?

Figure problems and postural conditions

Many clients are concerned about the distribution of their body fat which influences their shape. The most common problem in women is the rounded, heavy thighs, buttocks and hips commonly referred to as a 'pear-shape'. The therapist needs to assess the client fully and analyse whether the body fat is evenly distributed. They should also note any stretch marks and their cause, e.g. rapid weight loss or pregnancy, and the type of fat, e.g. cellulite, soft or hard. It is also important to build up a picture of the client's lifestyle, eating habits and dietary intake.

Soft fat
Soft fat is the easiest type of fat condition to mobilise. It is not firm and moves easily when touched. It is easy to manipulate and generally responds well to diet and exercise.

Hard fat
This type of fat is difficult to disperse and is firm to touch.

Cellulite
Cellulite is not a term that is recognised by the medical profession but it clearly exists and is not identifiable as any other fat type.

Cellulite affects mainly women and causes unsightly dimpling and puckering of the skin. It is normally found in the thigh and buttock areas. It gives a characteristic 'cool feel' to the skin as the blood circulation is diminished in the area. The formation of cellulite is linked to the female hormones, namely oestrogen and progesterone, which play a part in subcutaneous fat distribution. A person does not have to be overweight to be affected by cellulite. As well as being unattractive, cellulite can be painful as it can compress nerve endings. For these reasons, many women resort to the therapist for treatment. There are varying degrees of cellulite, namely hard and soft.

Stretch marks
Stretch marks, or striations as they are technically known, are caused by thinning and loss of elasticity in the dermis. On fair skins they first appear as red, raised lines becoming purple later on whereas on darker skins they initially appear as dark raised lines and eventually flatten to form shiny streaks usually between 6 and 12 mm long. They often occur on the hips and thighs during adolescent growth spurts and occur on approximately 75% of all pregnant women, especially on the abdomen and breast areas. It is for the latter reason that most women seek the advice of the therapist and providing they are caught in the early stages treatment can be effective. (See Chapter 7).

The two main reasons why stretch marks can occur are due to *endocrine cause* or *mechanical cause*.

It is known that corticosteroid hormones suppress fibre formation in the skin which in turn causes collagen found within the dermis to waste away. Consequently the organisation and texture of tissues is seriously affected and this can lead to a state of well defined marking of the skin. This is the endocrine cause of stretch marks.

It is thought that sudden and excessive weight increase does not allow the skin time to stretch gently, therefore 'ripping' of the collagen and elastin fibres occurs and leads to the appearance of stretch marks. This is a mechanical cause.

Figure and postural conditions

Deviation in body alignment can lead to a variety of figure and postural conditions, the main ones being outlined below.

Dowagers hump

This is a condition associated with old age. Fatty deposits build up at the back of the neck over a period of time as the client holds his/her head forward of the normal postural alignment.

Protruding abdomen

This often relates to the postural condition of lordosis. However it may also be the result of fatty deposits around the area or as result of weak abdominal muscles, a condition often found in post natal mothers.

Midriff bulge

This is a fairly common condition, often associated with the over 35 age group, where as a result of the ageing process, fatty deposits accumulate in this area. It tends to be more apparent in women than men.

Flat feet

Flat feet is a condition due to the absence or sinking of the medial longitudinal arch of the foot, caused by weakness of the ligaments and tendons.

Hallux valgus

Hallux valgus is a condition recognised by a deviation of the big toe from the mid-line. It is commonly referred to as a bunion.

Tibial torsion

Commonly referred to as 'knock knees', tibial torsion is generally due to a slack tendon supporting the knee. This enables the knees to rotate inwards towards the mid-line.

Winged scapulae

The shoulder blades protrude as they are adducted towards the mid line. This is a fairly common condition in back packers who carry heavy weights on their backs.

Round shoulders

Round shoulders are generally a result of the postural condition kyphosis. The pectoral muscles shorten creating a 'barrel chest'. Round shoulders are often associated with tall people who round their shoulders to appear smaller, ladies with large chests who try to conceal the size of their breasts and people suffering with severe asthma.

Kyphosis

Kyphosis may be recognised by the client's rounded shoulders. This shortens the pectoral muscles and curves the thoracic area of the vertebral column outwards. In women it can lead to sagging breasts as the suspensory ligaments and pectoral muscles normally hold the breasts upright. This condition is quite common in young girls with large breasts who through embarrassment curve their shoulders round to conceal themselves. It is also common in office workers, drivers and therapists whose everyday bodily posture involves rounding their shoulders.

Fig. 2.6 *Kyphosis*   **Fig. 2.7** *Lordosis*   **Fig. 2.8** *Scoliosis*

Lordosis

Lordosis is recognised by the hollow back created by the inward curvature of the lumbar area of the spinal column. The muscles of the back tighten and this often leads to back ache. In severe cases the pelvis tends to tilt forward, the abdomen and gluteals appear to protrude and the knees will hyper-extend, shortening the hamstrings in order to counter-balance the body weight. This condition is common in small people who often, through trying to appear taller, hollow out their backs. Gymnasts and ballet dancers can also suffer with this condition.

Scoliosis

Scoliosis is recognised by a lateral deviation of the vertebral column. The shortening of muscles on one side of the body can lead to dropped shoulders, uneven waist and scapulae and a tilting pelvis. Busy mothers who tend to hold their children on one side of their waist can suffer with scoliosis. Carrying heavy bags or standing with the body weight to one side can also lead to this condition.

POINT TO NOTE ▷ *Some spinal curvatures are structural and cannot be altered by the therapist.*

Postural assessment of the client

1 The therapist first assesses the client by observing their postural stance from a side view and notes any deviations to the points listed on p. 59–60.

Note. Whilst training it is common practice to use a weighted string (plumb line) as a guide to check that the body is in alignment or whether the client's head, shoulders, abdomen, pelvis, buttocks or knees are protruding forwards or behind the plumb line.

2 The therapist assesses the anterior then posterior view of the client.

Note. It is common practice whilst training for the trainee to:

* mark the individual vertebrae to see if there is any curvature of the spine
* mark the scapulae and measure the distance between them and the spine
* place their hands on either side of the waist to see if they are even
* place their hands on both shoulders to see if they are even.

3 The therapist observes the client's normal seating position noting the position of the head, shoulders, arms, waist, pelvis, legs, knees and feet.

4 The therapist notes the client's normal walking pattern, observing the gait of movement, the positioning of the skeleton and the distribution of body weight.

ACTIVITY

Perform a postural analysis on three different colleagues. Note your findings and research suitable corrective exercises for postural improvement.

POINT TO NOTE ▷ *The majority of postural conditions can be assisted by gentle corrective exercise undertaken by the client at home.*

Corrective exercise as home care advice

In order for the therapist to assist the client in gaining the maximum benefit from some salon treatments, e.g. neuro-muscular electrical stimulation, they need to have a basic understanding of the use of corrective exercise. A number of therapists develop an interest in exercise and take up specialist exercise courses which enable them to teach and fully advise on exercise programmes. There are also a great many books on types of exercises, mobility, muscle strength and fitness testing that would be useful further study.

Before advising any corrective exercises it is important to consider the:

* Age and mobility of the client.
* Muscle strength of the client.
* General health of the client
* Past history of exercise of the client.
* The environment in which the exercises will be carried out.

POINTS TO NOTE ▷
- *Youth does not always indicate that the fitness and mobility of a client are good.*
- *Muscle strength can be determined by testing through resistance-type exercises the strength of the client's muscles in different areas of the body.*
- *Exercise should not be performed for at least two hours after eating.*
- *Advise clients that they must not continue if they feel dizzy or if they feel any discomfort.*

Isotonic exercise

Isotonic exercise is a form of exercise that produces lengthening and shortening of the muscle fibres by movement of the joints, e.g. active exercise (exercise with movement).

Concentric and *eccentric* muscle work relates to isotonic exercise. Concentric is where the fibres, through shortening, become thicker, e.g. the biceps when the arm is bent. Eccentric is where the muscle fibres, through movement, lengthen, e.g. the triceps when the arm is bent.

Isometric exercise

Isometric exercise is exercise that causes the muscle fibres to contract without an overall change of length in the muscle, e.g. passive exercise (exercise without movement).

Corrective exercise

Corrective exercises may be recommended to supplement salon treatments providing the therapist is happy that there are no underlying medical conditions.

The normal pattern of exercise sequences would include warm-up exercises, aerobic exercises, strengthening and stretching exercises and a cool-down/relaxation period.

Warm-up exercises

Warm-up exercises prepare the body's physiology for action and so reduce the risk of injury. They should include:

- Mobility exercises (within the normal range of movement).
- General activity to gradually increase the heart and respiration rates and to stimulate circulation.
- Static stretches of the muscles to be exercised, held for 6–8 seconds.

Aerobic exercises

Aerobic exercises provide a sustained period of exercise at the correct level of intensity to increase the heart rate into the training zone. They should include:

- Build-up aerobics.
- Peak aerobics.
- Cool-down aerobics.

Strengthening and stretching exercises

Strengthening and stretching exercises are used to build up muscle strength and improve mobility. They can be used to correct postural conditions. Examples of exercises follow.

1 Arm lift – a strength exercise for kyphosis

Fig. 2.9 *Arm lift*

Purpose – To strengthen scapular adductors and help prevent or correct round shoulders and kyphosis.

Position – a Least difficult: lie prone with arms in reverse 'T'; forehead resting on floor.

– b More advanced: same as before except arms are extended overhead and held against the ears.

Movement – Maintain the arm position and contract the muscles between the shoulder blades, lifting the arms as high as possible without raising head and trunk. Hold, relax and repeat.

2 Wand exercise – a stretch exercise for kyphosis

Purpose – To help prevent and correct round shoulders and kyphosis by stretching the muscles on the anterior side of the shoulder joint.

Fig. 2.10 *Wand exercise*

Position – Sit with wand grasped at ends. Raise wand overhead. Be certain that the head does not slide forward into a 'poke neck' position. Keep the chin tucked and neck straight.

Movement – Bring the wand down behind the shoulder blades. Keep spine erect. Hold.
Hands may be moved closer together to increase stretch on chest muscles.

3   Pelvic tilt – a strength exercise for lordosis

Fig. 2.11   *Pelvic tilt*

Purpose – To strengthen the abdominals and help prevent or correct lumbar lordosis and backache.

Position – Supine with knees bent.

Movement – Tighten the abdominal muscles and tilt the pelvis backward; try to flatten the lower back against the floor. At the same time, tighten the hip and thigh muscles. Hold then relax. Breathe normally during the contraction, do not hold the breath.

4   Low back stretcher – a stretch exercise for lordosis

Purpose – To stretch hip flexors and lumbar muscles, and help prevent or correct lumbar lordosis and backache.

Fig. 2.12   *Low back stretcher*

67

Position – Supine position.

Movement – Draw one knee up to the chest and pull it down tightly with the hands, then slowly return it to the original position. Repeat with other knee. Do not grasp knee, but the thigh. If a partner or a weight stabilises the extended leg, the hip flexor muscles of that leg will also be stretched.

The therapist needs to advise on suitable exercises to stretch the shortened muscles and strengthen the lengthened muscles ensuring the starting position is appropriate to the client's mobility, muscle strength, balance and age range, e.g. an older client with unsteady balance would be more suited to exercises performed in a sitting position on a steady chair.

Isotonic and isometric exercises can be used and gradually, as muscle strength improves, resistance exercises using available home weights, e.g. jars of coffee, can be used to strengthen the arm muscles.

Cool-down/relaxation period
Cool down/relaxation exercises allow the body to cool down gradually and control breathing.

POINTS TO NOTE ▷
- *The types of exercise selected and the number of repetitions would vary according to the area being exercised and the mobility, strength and balance of the client.*
- *It is important to remind the client to continue breathing smoothly throughout exercise to maintain the intake of oxygen and exhalation of carbon dioxide.*
- *If the client's needs are greater than the therapist can offer, the therapist should recommend appropriate, qualified exercise specialists.*

PROGRESS CHECK

1 Describe how you would recognise the following conditions:
  a soft fat   c cellulite   e dowager's hump
  b hard fat   d stretch marks   f midriff bulge.

2 Explain what is meant by the following terms:
  a kyphosis   b lordosis   c scoliosis.

3 Before recommending corrective exercise home care advice what factors would you take into consideration?

4 Define the following terms:
  a isotonic exercise   c concentric muscle work
  b isometric exercise d eccentric muscle work.

Physical fitness

Every physical activity undertaken needs the body to produce energy from food digested and absorbed by the body. There are two systems which release energy from food; the *aerobic* system and the *anaerobic* system

The aerobic system provides energy for prolonged activity, i.e. for most activity. The anaerobic system provides energy for short periods of activity (up to ten seconds) and can be thought of as an 'emergency' system. The aerobic system utilises carbohydrates and fats to obtain energy whereas the anaerobic system utilises only carbohydrates. The body switches to the anaerobic system when the aerobic system cannot produce enough energy for the body's needs. Once the anaerobic system cannot produce enough energy, the body tires and needs to rest until waste products produced by the anaerobic system are removed. How well the aerobic and anaerobic systems work is one measure of physical fitness and is important for health.

Components of physical fitness may be classified as either health related components or skill related components.

Health related components of physical fitness are:

⊛ Cardiovascular fitness.

⊛ Muscular endurance.

⊛ Muscular strength.

⊛ Flexibility.

⊛ Body composition.

Skill related components of physical fitness are:

⊛ Agility.

⊛ Balance.

⊛ Co-ordination

⊛ Speed.

⊛ Power.

⊛ Reaction time.

GOOD PRACTICE ▷ *The therapist has a responsibility to constantly remind the client to take care when exercising if they have weak joints, poor posture, weak muscles or a bad back.*

Fig. 2.13 *Running in place*

Cardiovascular fitness

Cardiovascular fitness is a measure of the efficiency of the respiratory and circulatory systems. It is a term used to refer to how effectively oxygen is taken into the body and transported to the working muscles for energy and how effectively the waste produced is removed by the body.

A person who is considered to have a high cardio-respiratory endurance, i.e. they can exercise for a fair period of time at increased heart rate and recover reasonably fast, can be assumed to be 'aerobically fit'.

Exercise to test for cardiovascular fitness – running in place
Run in place for one and a half minutes (at a rate of 120 steps per minute). Rest for one minute and count the heart rate for thirty seconds. A heart rate of 60 or lower passes.

Examples of aerobic activity, i.e. activity that improves cardiovascular fitness, are jogging, swimming, brisk walking and aerobics.

Muscular endurance

This refers to the individual's ability to repeatedly use the same muscle or muscles without getting tired. Many athletes display high muscular endurance, e.g. swimmers and long distance runners.

Exercise to test for muscular endurance – side leg raise

Fig. 2.14 *Side leg raise*

Lie on the floor on your side. Lift your leg up and to the side of the body until your feet are 24–36 inches apart. Hold for as long as possible. Perform 10 repetitions with each leg.

Isometric examples of muscular endurance exercises are; gluteal squeeze, pelvic tilt, arm press.

Isotonic examples of muscular endurance exercises are; squats, curl ups, back extensions.

Muscular strength

Muscular strength describes the amount of force an individual muscle or group of muscles can produce in overcoming a resistance in one maximum voluntary contraction, e.g. lifting a heavy weight.

Muscular strength can be tested by using dynamometers or manual tests for different parts of the body, e.g. press ups for the arms and chest.

Exercise to test muscular strength – press ups

Fig. 2.15 *Press ups*

USEFUL INFORMATION

Full press ups may be a muscular strength exercise to some individuals but an endurance exercise to others depending upon their strength.

70

Lie face down on the floor. Place the hands under the shoulders. Keeping the legs and body straight, press off the floor until the arms are fully extended. Women repeat once, men three times.

Examples of muscular strength exercises are press ups and exercises done with variable resistance machines and free weights.

Flexibility

Flexibility can be measured by a person's range of movement. Flexibility will actually determine how an athlete can perform, as if muscles are tight and joints are inflexible, agility, range of movement, balance and speed are all restricted.

Exercise for testing flexibility of the hamstrings and lower back – toe touch

Fig. 2.16 *Toe touch*

Sit on the floor with your feet against a wall. Keep the feet together and the knees straight. Bend forward at the hips. Reach forward and touch your closed fists to the wall. Bend forward slowly, do not bounce.

a Triceps   b Adductors   c Obliques

Fig. 2.17 *Examples of flexibility exercises*

71

Body composition

The composition of a person's body refers to the relative percentages of muscle, fat, bone and other tissues that make up the body. It can be thought of as a measure of whether a person is under or over weight, i.e. has a low or high percentage of body fat.

Body composition can be measured by using calibrated skin callipers. Four measurements are taken from different parts of the body. These measurements are then compared with a chart of accepted norms and an estimate of the percentage of body fat read off. This test can also be performed manually.

Fig. 2.18 *Measuring body composition*

Manual measurement of body composition – the pinch

Have a partner pinch a fold of skin on the back of your upper arm halfway between the tip of the elbow and the tip of the shoulder. Measurements of 1 inch for men and $1\frac{1}{2}$ inches for women are acceptable.

Agility

Agility is the ability to rapidly and accurately change the direction of the entire body in space. Examples of sports that require agility are skiing and wrestling.

Balance

Balance is the maintenance of equilibrium whilst stationary or moving. Balance is very important in gymnastic beam exercises and water skiing

Co-ordination

Co-ordination is a person's ability to use the senses, e.g. sight and hearing, in conjunction with the body parts to perform motor tasks smoothly and accurately. Good co-ordination is needed for golf.

Speed

Speed is the ability to perform a movement in a short period of time, e.g. running.

Power

Power is a person's ability to transfer energy into force at a fast rate. Discus throwing requires power.

Reaction time

A person's reaction time is the time elapsed between stimulation and the beginning of reaction to that stimulation, e.g. from starting block to sprint take-off.

Fitness testing

Before anyone undertakes an exercise regime in a professionally supervised leisure club or gym it is usual, after their initial consultation, that they be given a test to establish their level of fitness. A fitness test is used to assess where an individual's strengths and weaknesses lie, to meet the perceived needs of the client and to prevent injury.

Tests vary in their degree of sophistication depending upon the requirement of the client. Such tests should include measurements of:

- Height and weight.
- Peak flow.
- Cardiovascular fitness.
- Body composition, i.e. percentage body fat.

Conclusions are reached on an individual's fitness by comparing test results against accepted norms related to age, sex and body type.

ACTIVITY   Perform tests to identify a client's level of cardiovascular fitness, muscular strength and endurance and flexibility.

POINTS TO NOTE ▷
- *Every exercise if not performed correctly is potentially dangerous.*
- *Muscular strength and endurance exercises are usually combined.*
- *Breathing should be natural throughout exercise.*

Considerations for safe exercise

All the following should be taken into consideration when assessing whether exercise at a particular level is safe for a client:

- Heart conditions; high blood pressure; dizziness.
- Severe respiratory conditions; asthma.
- Fever.
- Recent operations.
- Broken bones.

* Other medical conditions such as diabetes, epilepsy and pregnancy.
* Whether the client has eaten a heavy meal or consumed alcohol.

Always remember that every exercise if not performed correctly is potentially dangerous!

ACTIVITY

Devise a suitable exercise plan for:

a a 50 year old female client with lordosis

b 30 year old female office worker with kyphosis

c 40 year old postman with scoliosis.

Name	Date
Address	
Tel. no.	
Date of birth	
Medical history	
High blood pressure	Medication
Asthma	Number of pregnancies
Dizziness/fainting	Ages of children
Anaemia	
Weight	Frame size
Height	% Body fat

Reason for exercise:

Lose fat( )   Change appearance( )   Gain strength( )   Feel fitter( )   Sports performance( )

Doctors advice( )   Social( )   Other

Fig. 2.19 *Example of an exercise consultation card*

PROGRESS CHECK

1 Explain the difference between the aerobic and anaerobic systems.

2 Describe the following components of health-related fitness:
 a cardiovascular fitness   d flexibility
 b muscular strength   e body composition.
 c muscular endurance

3 Explain the different components of skill-related fitness.

4 State the considerations for safe exercise.

5 List the points that should be noted on an exercise consultation card.

KEY TERMS

You need to know what these words and phrases mean. Go back through the chapter to find out.

Nutrition	Vitamins	Good posture
Proteins	Metabolism	Isotonic and
Carbohydrates	Basal metabolism	isometric exercise
Fats	Types of diets	Components of
Roughage	Eating problems	fitness
Mineral elements	Body types	

3 Health, safety, reception, stock control and consultation

After working through this chapter you will be able to:

➤ list different types of infections and infestations

➤ carry out emergency procedures

➤ describe the activities undertaken in the reception area

➤ deal with telephone messages

➤ make a number of appointments for clients

➤ understand the purpose of stock control

➤ explain the purpose of a consultation

➤ carry out an effective facial and body consultation

Hygiene

It is paramount that the therapist ensures the highest standards of hygiene within the salon. Because of the close proximity of therapist and client good hygiene is essential to prevent infection, cross infection and infestation.

Protecting against disease

We spend a great deal of our lives surrounded by what are commonly known as 'germs'. Some germs are harmless, some are even beneficial, but others present a danger to us because they cause disease.

The germs which cause disease are usually spread by:

● Unclean hands.

● Contaminated tools.

● Sores and pus.

● Discharges from the nose and mouth.

● Shared use of items such as towels and cups.

● Close contact with infected skin cells.

● Contaminated blood or tissue fluid.

Viruses

Viruses are the tiniest germs, yet they are responsible for an enormous range of human diseases. Viruses can only survive in living cells. The following are examples of viral infections:

● **Common cold**: the virus is spread by coughing and sneezing and is carried through the air as a droplet infection.

* **Herpes simplex** (cold sores): the virus remains dormant in the mucous membranes of the skin. It can be activated by sunlight or general debility. Cold sores are most likely to spread when they are weeping.
* **Warts**: there are several types of wart. Verruca plantaris is a wart which occurs commonly on the soles of the feet and is spread by close contact.

Bacteria

Bacteria are single-celled organisms. They grow from spores which are very resistant to attack and multiply very quickly. Bacteria are capable of breeding outside the body and can therefore be caught easily through personal contact or by touching a contaminated article.

Fig. 3.1 A typical bacterial cell

Some bacteria cause diseases and infect wounds. The following are examples of bacterial infections:

* **Impetigo**: bacteria enter the body through broken skin and cause blisters which weep and crust over. The condition is highly infectious and can be spread easily by dirty tools.
* **Boils**: these can occur when bacteria invade the hair follicle through a surface scratch or by close contact with an infected person.
* **Whitlow**: this can be caused by the bacteria invading the pad of the finger through a break in the skin which has often been caused by a splinter.

Fungi

Fungi are yeasts and moulds. Moulds break down all sorts of materials but rarely cause disease. Yeasts are single-celled fungi which can cause disease. Fungal infections are very easily transmitted by personal contact or by touching contaminated articles. The following are examples of fungal infections:

* **Tinea pedis** (athletes foot): the fungus thrives in the warm, moist environment between the toes and sometimes on the soles of the feet. The condition is picked up easily by direct contact with recently shed, infected skin cells.
* **Tinea unguium** (ringworm of the nail): may result from contact with the fungus present on other parts of the body, e.g. toenails may become infected during an outbreak of athletes foot, which if touched could then be spread by contact to the nails.

Animal parasites

Animal parasites are small insects which cause disease by invading the skin and using human blood or protein as a source of nourishment. Diseases caused by animal parasites usually occur as the result of prolonged contact with an infected person. The following are examples of diseases caused by animal parasites:

* **Scabies**: tiny mites burrow through the outside layer of the epidermis and lay their eggs underneath the skin surface. The condition is very itchy and causes a rash and swelling. Characteristic line formations show where the burrows have been formed.

* **Head lice**: small parasites which puncture the skin and suck blood. They lay eggs on the hair close to the scalp. The unhatched eggs are called *nits* and can be seen as shiny, pearl-coloured, oval bodies which cling to the hair shaft.

To protect against the spread of disease you must:

* Provide each client with clean towels and gown.

* Carry out a consultation before each treatment to ensure contra-indications are spotted in time.

* Use only tools which have been cleaned and sterilised.

* Use correct treatment techniques to avoid injuring the client.

* Dispose of waste properly after each treatment.

* Wash your own hands before each treatment and as necessary throughout the treatment.

* Maintain high standards of personal hygiene.

GOOD PRACTICE ▷

* *Dirt and bacteria accumulate in cracks. You must not use tools with a damaged edge as they cannot be sterilised effectively.*

* *You have a responsibility to yourself, your clients and your colleagues to always work hygienically and to do everything you can to avoid the spread of infection.*

* *All work surfaces should be cleaned regularly with hot water and detergent. The treatment couch, trolley, sink and stools should be wiped down at the end of each working day with a solution of disinfectant.*

* *Waste should not be handled or exposed. Make sure that the waste resulting from your treatments is placed in a lined container, tied up and disposed of in a large sealed refuse sack with other salon waste.*

ACTIVITY

Research the different skin conditions caused by bacterial, viral and fungal infections. Note their names and characteristics.

Sterilisation and disinfection

Sterilisation is the destruction of all living organisms. It is very difficult to maintain sterile conditions. Once sterilised items have been exposed to the air they are no longer sterile. Articles which have been sterilised and stored hygienically for a short period are safe to use on the client.

Fig. 3.2 *Autoclave*

Autoclave

The most effective method of sterilisation is steaming at high pressure in an autoclave. This works on exactly the same principle as a pressure cooker. Steam is produced from a reservoir of water and is contained under pressure at a minimum of 121°C for 15 minutes. Modern autoclaves have thermochromic indicators which change colour when the required temperature has been reached. Stainless steel and glass items are suitable for sterilisation by this method. A stacking facility is usually provided so that the articles can be placed at different levels in the autoclave. The temperatures used in autoclaves vary from 121°C to 134°C and with correct time and heat exposure kill all spores. However the range of temperature can affect certain materials, e.g. soft plastics.

POINT TO NOTE ▷ It is recommended by the Health and Safety Executive that autoclaves should have dials for temperature and pressure.

Sanitisers

Sanitisers operate by irradiating implements with ultra-violet light. This would normally inactivate any bacteria, but as all implements cannot be fully exposed directly to the ultra-violet light, these units are now only recommended for storage of sterilised implements.

Fig. 3.3 *Sanitiser*

POINTS TO NOTE ▷ • The ultra-violet light is at its strongest directly underneath the lamp and weaker at the front of the unit.
• Shaded areas of implements, such as the blades of scissors, receive no exposure to the ultra-violet light.

Glass bead sterilisers

Glass bead sterilisers reach temperatures between 190 and 300°C (374–572°F) depending on the model. This temperature has to be maintained for 30-60 minutes prior to use. If extra items are put into the steriliser

Fig. 3.4 *Glass bead steriliser*

during this period, the temperature of the beads drops and the effects are lost. Timing has to begin again. Glass bead sterilisers can hold only very small items, e.g. tweezers, and therefore have limited use in the salon.

Chemical methods of sterilisation

Concentrated liquid chemical agents are available which have to be diluted for use. Some chemical agents act as a sterilant, depending on the strength of the solution and the time for which items are kept in contact with them. Some liquid chemical sterilisers are very harmful to the skin and great care is needed when handling them.

Fig. 3.5 *Chemical sterilisation equipment*

GOOD PRACTICE ▷ *You must be sure that you are carrying out safe and effective hygienic procedures. Always read and follow manufacturers instructions carefully when preparing, using and disposing of chemical solutions.*

Disinfection

Disinfectants work against bacteria and fungi, but they just remove contamination; they do not necessarily kill spores. Disinfectants only reduce the number of organisms. Examples of good chemical disinfectants are:

* **Gluteraldehyde**: a 2% solution is used which remains active for 14–18 days, after which time it must be discarded. Gluteraldehyde is particularly useful for soaking metal instruments and applicators, but must be handled with great care. (See COSHH, Chapter 11.)

* **Alcohol**: alcohol disinfectants have a very effective bactericidal effect. They must be used once only and then discarded.

* **Quartery ammonium compounds**: these are bacteriostatic cleansing agents. They prevent bacteria from spreading but are not effective against very resistant organisms.

* **Hypochlorites**: these products contain sodium or calcium hypochlorite and are often used for general cleaning purposes as they are relatively cheap. Some are corrosive and should not be used for soaking metal instruments.

POINT TO NOTE ▷ *Quartery ammonium compounds are inactivated by soap.*

GOOD PRACTICE ▷
* *Tools should always be washed in warm soapy water and rinsed well in clean water before disinfecting or sterilising them. This ensures the removal of debris which would act as a barrier. It also prevents contamination of the soaking solution.*
* *The risks of cross infection will only be eliminated if potential disease is identified, immediate measures taken and tools and equipment are kept scrupulously clean throughout the treatment.*

Antiseptics

Antiseptics are disinfectants used specifically on the skin and for treating wounds. Ready-for-use swabs impregnated with 70% isopropyl alcohol are often used for convenience.

POINT TO NOTE ▷ *Aseptic conditions refer to creating an environment which will avoid infection.*

ACTIVITY

Research the different cleaning and sterilising methods used in two salons. Make a note of any special instructions on diluting, using and disposing of the chemical disinfectants and sterilising agents used.

Emergency first aid

You need a basic knowledge of first aid so that you can assist with minor accidental injuries or unexpected situations which happen from time to time in the salon. More serious injuries, for example those involving acute pain or loss of consciousness or serious bleeding, should be dealt with by a qualified first aider, doctor or nurse.

First aid kit

The Health and Safety regulations require the salon to have a first aid kit readily available. The contents are specified and are intended to cover most emergency situations.

The first aid kit must include:
* A first aid guidance card
* Assorted plasters (preferably waterproof)

81

- Different sizes of sterile dressings
- Bandages
- Sterile eye pads
- Scissors
- Tweezers
- Safety pins.

Useful additions to this list are:

- Surgical adhesive tape
- Antiseptic cleansing products, i.e. liquid and cream
- An eye bath
- Gauze
- Crepe bandages
- An antihistamine cream
- Medical wipes
- Cotton wool.

If the salon has a fridge with a freezer compartment it is a good idea to keep an ice pack for injuries which produce swelling.

It is advisable to keep a stock of disposable gloves to wear when dealing with open wounds. These give some protection from hepatitis B and AIDS if an infection is present.

All staff should know what the first aid box looks like and where it is kept. It is recommended that the box is green with a white cross marked on it and that it is dustproof and free from damp.

Fig. 3.6 First aid kit

GOOD PRACTICE ▷ • *Contaminated cotton wool and dressings should be disposed of in a plastic bag which has been tied up.*

⊛ All accidents which occur in the salon must be recorded in an accident register. This is a requirement of the Health and Safety at Work Act.

⊛ Keep in the first aid box a card which lists names, addresses and phone numbers of the local health centres and hospitals.

Table 3.1 First aid situations the therapist may have to deal with

Problem	Priority	Action
Minor cuts	To stop the bleeding	Apply pressure over cotton wool taking care to avoid contact with the blood.
Severe cuts	To stop the bleeding	Keep applying pressure over a clean towel until qualified help arrives. Put on disposable gloves as soon as possible.
Electric shock	To remove from source of electricity	Do not touch the person until they are disconnected from the electricity supply. If breathing has stopped, artificial respiration will need to be given by a qualified person. Ring for an ambulance.
Dizziness	To restore the flow of blood to the head	Position the person with their head down between their knees and loosen their clothing.
Fainting	To restore the flow of blood to the head	Lie the person down with their feet raised on a cushion.
Nose bleed	To constrict the flow of blood	Sit the client up with the head bent forward. Loosen the clothing around the neck. Pinch the soft part of the nose firmly until bleeding has stopped. Make sure breathing continues through the mouth during this period. If bleeding has not stopped after half an hour, medical attention must be sought.
Burns	To cool the skin and prevent it from breaking	Hold the affected area under cold, running water until the pain is relieved. Serious burns should be covered loosely with a sterile dressing and medical attention sought.
Epilepsy	To prevent self-injury and relieve embarrassment	Do not interfere forcibly with a person during an attack. Gently prevent them from injuring themselves. Ensure the person's airways are clear and wipe away any froth which forms at the mouth. After the attack, cover with a blanket, comfort and give reassurance until recovery is complete.
Objects in the eye	To remove the object without damaging the eye	Expose the invaded area and try stroking the object towards the inside corner of the eye with a dampened twist of cotton wool. If this is not successful, help the person to use an eye bath containing clean warm water.
Falls	To determine if there is spine damage. To treat minor injuries if the fall is not serious	If the person complains of pains in the back or neck, then do not move them: cover with a warm blanket and get medical aid immediately. For less serious falls, treat the bruises, cuts, sprains or grazes as appropriate.

Table 3.1 *First aid situations the therapist may have to deal with (continued)*

Problem	Priority	Action
Bruises	To reduce pain and swelling	Apply cold compresses for 30 minutes using a towel wrapped round an ice-pack or very cold tap water. Keep the compress in place with a bandage. Replace it if it dries out.
Grazes	To clean wound and prevent infection	Soak a pad of cotton wool with an antiseptic and gently clean the graze, working outwards from the centre. Replace the cotton wool regularly throughout the cleaning. Apply a sterile gauze dressing, preferably a non-adherent type, to protect the wound as it heals. If dirt or foreign matter has become embedded in the graze, the person should be referred to a doctor who may want to give a tetanus injection.
Sprains	To reduce swelling	Apply cold compresses to the area (see treatment for bruises) and support the affected joint with a bandage firmly applied. Refer the person to a doctor.

AIDS (Acquired Immune Deficiency Syndrome)

Aids is caused by the human immuno-deficiency virus (HIV). The virus attacks the body's natural immune system and makes it very vulnerable to other infections which eventually cause death. Some people are known to be HIV positive, which means that they are carrying the virus without the symptoms of AIDS. HIV carriers are able to pass on the virus to someone else through infected blood or tissue fluid, for example through cuts or broken skin. The virus does not live for long outside the body.

Hepatitis B

This is a disease of the liver is caused by a virus (HBV) which is transmitted by infected blood and tissue fluids. The virus is very resistant and can survive outside the body. People can be very ill for a long time with a hepatitis B infection. It is a very weakening disease which can be fatal.

Strict hygiene practices are essential to prevent hepatitis B from spreading in the salon.

POINT TO NOTE ▷ *It is important to protect against all diseases which are carried by blood and tissue fluids. Many people feel most threatened by AIDS: this is mainly because of intense media pressure, during 1993–4, which emphasised the high mortality rate. In fact there is a much higher risk of cross-infection with hepatitis B, because the HBV virus is so resistant and can survive outside the body.*

ACTIVITY

With a colleague role play emergency first aid procedures for each of the following:

a nose bleed

b dizziness

c object in the eye

d fainting.

PROGRESS CHECK

1 Give an example of each of the following types of infection:

   a viral   **b** bacterial   **c** fungal   **d** animal parasite.

2 Define the following:

   a sterilisation   **b** disinfection   **c** antiseptic.

3 Explain why it is advisable to wear protective gloves when treating an open wound.

4 State the first aid treatment for a client suffering with:

   a a burn   **b** a nose bleed   **c** an epileptic fit.

Reception

The reception is the central pivot for the staff and clients of the salon. It is an area that everyone has to walk through either as a member of staff entering work, greeting clients or as a client when making and waiting for appointments. Everybody's day revolves around the salon's appointment schedule, and therefore the reception area.

Fig. 3.7 *Reception*

First impressions do count so it is paramount that the reception area is inviting to the client. Therapeutic music rather than a loud, thudding pop record will aid relaxation for the majority of clients, and the use of essential oils either through burners or fans can saturate the air with a pleasant aroma. The seating should be comfortable in order to allow the client to begin to relax prior to treatment. The decor should reflect the type of premises and clientele the salon is marketing itself to, it should be continually refreshed to keep it in pristine condition and should be kept clean and tidy:

- All surfaces should be dusted and cleaned and waste bins should be emptied on a regular basis.
- Cups and glasses should be removed as soon as possible after use.
- Salon leaflets should be replaced before they become torn or out of date.

GOOD PRACTICE ▷

- *The reception is the ideal area to market you and your salon as you have a captive audience. Instead of purchasing magazines which advertise commercial skin care products produce regular salon leaflets which advertise you, your salon and the professional products you retail.*
- *Emphasise a healthy lifestyle by displaying information on diet and exercise.*
- *Serve healthy drinks to your clients, e.g. mineral water and fruit juices rather than only caffeine drinks such as coffee and tea.*
- *Reference materials should be presented in an attractive but practical manner to withstand regular reading, etc.*

The receptionist

Some establishments employ a receptionist, in others the therapists share the responsibility. The receptionist is the first point of contact clients and visitors have with the salon. It is therefore essential that the receptionist has a thorough understanding of the workings of the establishment and is extremely professional in their approach and appearance. It is also beneficial if the receptionist has an understanding of the benefits of the treatments and retail products on offer in the salon.

Many employers are fully aware of the benefits of offering retail products to their staff at cost price together with ensuring that they have experienced all of the salon treatments on offer to the clients as well as having treatments to benefit their individual needs. The image of the salon is reflected by the appearance of the staff. Just think when was the last time you saw a sales assistant in a top fashion retail outlet dressed in scruffy clothes?

POINT TO NOTE ▷ *It is useful for therapists to have treatments in the salon and role play the treatment as a realistic client, noting the way the reception area looked and how the receptionist and therapist interacted with them and each other.*

The reception area is the life-line of the salon. It is here that:

* The appointment book is kept. This is the central control of the salon, everybody plans their activities for the day around this.
* Appointments are made either by telephone or in person.
* Clients are greeted and made welcome by the receptionist.
* Clients and visitors to the salon, e.g. cosmetic company representatives, are taken care of whilst waiting. (It is extremely important, however, that staff do not discuss any business matters in an area where clients may overhear financial purchasing arrangements, etc.)
* Enquiries are dealt with, e.g. information on salon treatments, products, planned salon events, directions to another shop in the area.
* Products are ordered, received, recorded, priced, displayed and sold.
* Salon services are advertised.
* Payment is taken for treatments and retail products.

All of the tasks outlined above are generally undertaken by the receptionist, whose job role mainly involves taking, receiving and recording information either by telephone or in person.

Dealing with clients, visitors and reception enquiries

In order for a receptionist to deal either with clients or visitors to the salon they need to fully understand the workings of the salon including the:

* Roles and responsibilities of each member of staff.
* Recording mechanisms of the salon.
* Treatments offered by the salon and their benefits.
* Retail products sold by the salon.

The receptionist must remain courteous to all clients and visitors and treat them all as equals. Generally clients are polite and friendly, however some people can demand a great deal of attention and at times be aggressive and rude. The receptionist must stay cool, calm and collected; she represents the salon and as the first point of contact will create an impression of the salon to the client or visitor. A friendly smile and voice can often help to calm an aggressive visitor. We all have bad days, but when working in a service industry our moods have to be left at home. Clients and visitors may not always manage to do this so remember that you are probably just an outlet for their emotions, it is likely that it isn't personal and shouldn't be taken as such.

POINT TO NOTE ▷ *Behaviour breeds behaviour. Remember the last time your brother or sister shouted at you? You probably shouted back, next time try smiling and responding in a quiet calm voice until they are softened by your behaviour.*

Telephone enquiries

For many clients the telephone is their contact with the business. A good receptionist never forgets that all calls are from individuals and that each one of them is a prospective client.

You should always:

* Answer promptly – on the second or third ring. This gives both sides time to prepare themselves without the caller becoming impatient.
* Be friendly – give the name of the salon and say who you are. Note the client's name so that you can use it in the conversation.
* Smile when you pick up the receiver. Smiles definitely do travel down the telephone!
* Be enthusiastic – ask how you may help the caller. Enthusiasm is infectious and shows you enjoy being helpful.
* Listen attentively – it is very off-putting for a caller if they sense you are being distracted by someone else.
* Leave a good impression. Remember that you are the salon to the caller. Repeat back to them any important points discussed and thank them for calling. Don't forget to use their name!

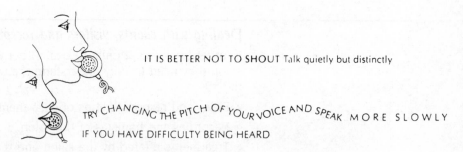

IT IS BETTER NOT TO SHOUT Talk quietly but distinctly

TRY CHANGING THE PITCH OF YOUR VOICE AND SPEAK MORE SLOWLY IF YOU HAVE DIFFICULTY BEING HEARD

Fig. 3.8 *Tips for using the telephone*

POINTS TO NOTE ▷

* *The salon telephone is for business and should not be used for chatty personal calls. Clients who cannot get through may give up and make an appointment somewhere else.*
* *It is a good idea for a salon to have a telephone answering machine. This records messages outside business hours and is particularly useful for clients to use in the event of a cancellation.*

Taking messages

It is essential that all messages are accurately recorded and promptly dealt with. The receptionist or therapist must ensure they record who the message is for, who it is from, the telephone number where the caller can be contacted, the date and time of the message and the actual message and state whether the caller wants their call returned, will call again or was returning a call. The person taking the message should also record

To: Date:

From: Time:

Tel. no.:   Taken by:

Message:

Please return their call

Will call again

Returning your call

MAKE SURE ALL INFORMATION IS CLEARLY RECORDED AND PASSED ON PROMPTLY.

Fig. 3.9   *Message recording sheet*

their own name in case there are any queries. An example of a message recording sheet is shown in Fig. 3.9.

Recording appointments

Recording appointments is an extremely important part of the receptionist's job and it is essential that all staff understand the appointment system that the salon operates. Appointment sheets are always made up in advance thus enabling clients to book courses of treatments.

The receptionist has to:

● Ensure that the reception desk is supplied with appointment cards, pens, pencils, ruler and rubber.

● Prepare pages in the appointment book at least six weeks in advance, to show the availability of each therapist on a particular day.

● As appointments are arranged, transfer the details to the appointment book in pencil, stating the client's name, their telephone number and the treatment required.

● Make out an appointment card for the client, recording details in pen and stating the date, day, time, therapist's name and treatment booked.

● Check the accuracy of both sets of records before handing over the appointment card to the client.

● Record the client's arrival at the salon by drawing a diagonal line in pencil across their details in the appointment book.

● When the client has gone through for treatment, draw a diagonal line across the first one to record that they are being attended to.

Clients who arrive unexpectedly may be treated provided that there is a therapist available. The receptionist should always check first and then record the client's details on the day in the appointment book.

DATE Monday..October...17th   COMPLEXION

	LOREEN	SAIDA	LIZ	JEAN	PAUL	SUNBED
8.30						
8.45						
9.00	Ms. Warner		Miss Williams	Mrs Lacey GTS		Mrs Turvey C
9.15	Super	Mrs Cogin		705 7997		646 2216
9.30	Cathio		AHA	Mrs Farmer		Miss Bates
9.45			424 5780	Cellulite treat		777 3454
10.00	221 4477	BODY	Mrs Rees	292 3987	Morning off	Ms. Faulkner
10.15		WRAP	Ultratone	Mrs Peet		273 2727 DNA
10.30			252 3790	Massage		Miss Laidlaw
10.45	Mrs Perry	707 2700	Mrs Christopher			827 1343
11.00	Dynatone		Back massage 551 9829	499 2000		Mr Cartwright
11.15	417 9173	Mrs Loy	Mrs Cooke	Mrs Dowding		266 0479
11.30	Ms. Harris	Massage	Massage	Dynatone		
11.45	Massage					
12.00		303 2768	448 4790	550 4171		Mr Burke
12.15	335 3939	Mrs Fabes		Miss Lulham		324 1567
12.30		Dynatone	LUNCH		Mr Ashford	Mrs Wensley
12.45	LUNCH	923 5625		Super Cathio	Massage	417 9894
13.00		Ms. Puttick				Ms Sullivan
13.15		Ultratone	Mrs Walker	217 9239	842 9111	344 3916
13.30		292 7652	AHA		Mr Lakin Back Massage 978 3493	Mrs Godfrey 237 8999
13.45	Mrs Turner					
14.00	Massage	LUNCH	506 4455	LUNCH	Mr Ward Massage	Mrs Bona 462 3911
14.15						
14.30					320 3493	Ms. C Bailey 121 3790

	Available Time		Client has been taken for treatment
	Client arrived and is awaiting treatment	DNA	Did Not Attend - Client did not inform: make a note on record card
		C	Last minute cancellation

Fig. 3.10 *Example of a completed page of an appointment book*

In some salons the receptionist prepares a list for each therapist which shows their schedule for the day. This is kept by the therapist and provides a useful quick reference.

GOOD PRACTICE ▷
- It is important that the appointment pages are kept neat and tidy. The correct codes and abbreviations must be used and the start and finish times of treatments made clear.
- Sometimes clients have to cancel or change their appointment. When details are recorded in pencil, they can be rubbed out neatly and the space used for another client.

ACTIVITY

1 Undertake reception duties and keep a log of all the tasks involved.
2 Monitor a colleague undertaking reception duties and identify their strengths along with any areas they need to improve upon. Record the information and present it clearly and logically.
3 With a group of colleagues role play a receptionist, therapist and a client (pleasant and difficult). Video the scenes, analyse and record the receptionist's behaviour highlighting their strengths and weaknesses.

Maintaining stock and the retail area

In many salons stock taking and ordering are undertaken by the receptionist. However it may be a task given to a therapist or the salon manager. It is extremely important that retail products are accessible and a good stock level is maintained or sales could be lost.

If the receptionist is responsible for the salon's stock they must:

* Keep the retail area clean and tidy: the counter, shelves and stock should be dusted every day and where possible have regular changes of display. Stock which is grubby and dusty will lose its value.
* Inform clients of current promotions: the receptionist should draw special offers to the attention of the clients and make sure the promotional material is displayed where it will catch the client's eye.
* Carry out stock checks: stock checks should be carried out weekly to monitor how well different products are selling and to make sure that popular lines are re-ordered before being sold out.
* Price the retail products: identical products must not be priced differently. Price tickets should be checked as part of regular stock checks. Old price tickets should be removed before putting on new ones so that a lower price is not disguised.
* Store stock correctly so that that it does not deteriorate or become damaged. Keep fast-moving lines at the front of the shelves and slower moving ones nearer the back. Do not block aisles or passageways with containers of stock; keep it in a locked cupboard or secure room.
* Display stock attractively: displays should be set up with the minimum disruption to business. If all retail stock is to be displayed, extra space is needed for the fastest selling lines. Shelving should be clean, safe and undamaged and strong enough to take the weight of the products on display. Packaging should be displayed with the product. Take care with flimsy packaging and stack heavier goods lower down than more fragile items.
* Keep accurate stock records. The quality of a product cannot be guaranteed once its expiry date has passed. Stock which has been stored beyond its 'shelf-life' has either to be sold off cheaply or, ideally, disposed of.
* Store stock in a cool, dark place.

┌ USEFUL INFORMATION ┐

Storing stock in straight lines makes counting easier.

91

Fig. 3.11 *Correct lifting and carrying technique; avoid straining your back when moving heavy items*

- Do not pile boxes too high.
- When an order arrives, bring old stock to the front and store new stock behind. This method of stock control is called FIFO, i.e. first in, first out.

POINTS TO NOTE ▷

- *Use dummy stock under bright lighting: this way the colour, texture and fragrance of the products will not become spoiled.*
- *Be careful when unpacking stock. Look out for sharp staple fastenings on boxes and avoid using a knife. Protect your overall when carrying large items. Paper and cardboard packages should be flattened before disposal.*
- *The salon loses money on old stock which is sold off cheaply or thrown away. Products which are approaching their expiry date should be identified at the stock check and steps taken to sell them before its too late. This may mean offering a special promotion or reducing the price slightly as an incentive to buy.*
- *Take care when dismantling a display. Put back equipment where it will not become damaged and keep tools and accessories safe in a box.*

The stock sheet lists the number of items in stock per product line. The details of a stock check are recorded on a stock sheet before being transferred to the stock book.

The stock book identifies reorder levels, and the receipt and sales of stock.

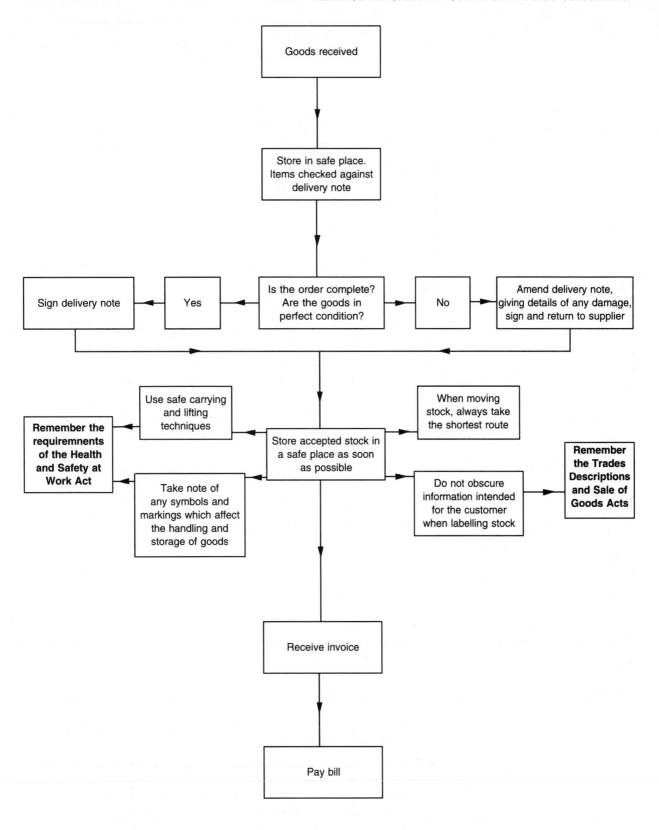

Fig. 3.12 *Distribution of stock*

	Stock List	
1	Aromatic oil for vapouriser or steam cabinet	30ml
2	Aromatic oil for body massage	30ml
3	Desincrustation gel	250g
4	Ionto gel DS	250g
5	Ionto gel GS	250g
6	Ionto gel SS	250g
7	Ionto gel DC	250g
8		
9		
10		

Fig. 3.13 *Example of a stock sheet*

No.	PRODUCT CODE	PRODUCT	STOCK LEVEL		Date 19/6/95							Date 20/6/95						
			Min	Max	COUNTER STOCK	STOCK ROOM STOCK	TOTAL STOCK (I)	ORDER	RECIEVED	TOTAL STOCK (II)	SOLD	COUNTER STOCK	STOCK ROOM STOCK	TOTAL STOCK (I)	ORDER	RECIEVED	TOTAL STOCK (II)	SOLD
1	00070	Aromatic oil for vap/sc 30ml	10	14	6	2	8	2	–	8	–	6	2	8	–	2	10	–
2	00071	Cellulite cream 150g	6	8	3	3	6	2	–	6	2	3	1	4	2	2	6	1
3	000072	Stretch mark cream	6	8	4	4	8	–	–	8	1	3	4	7	–	–	7	–
4	000073																	
5	00074																	
6	00075																	

Fig. 3.14 *Example of a stock book*

GOOD PRACTICE

- *Ensure a good system of stock control is implemented highlighting the item, size and minimum and maximum levels of stock required.*
- *Review stock control system regularly as requirements may fluctuate due to factors such as: the time of year, promotions and changes in current trends. Seek advice from your product supplier who will have experience of these. They may also provide you with a useful stock control system.*
- *Ensure stock is available or sales will be lost!*

ACTIVITY

With a colleague, discuss the following and compare your answers with other members of your group:

a What could be the possible reasons for discrepancies at a stock check?

b How do you think that seasonal variations might affect the allocation of space given to stock?

c When are the best times for changing displays and attending to stock?

d Why should the salon aim for a fast turnover of stock?

e What sort of things should be considered when fitting out a stock room.

PROGRESS CHECK

1 List the roles of a receptionist.

2 Describe how the reception can be used for marketing.

3 List the important points that should be noted when taking a telephone message.

4 State why pencils are often used to record information in the appointment book.

5 Give the reasons for carrying out regular stock checks.

6 What is the main purpose of:
   a a stock sheet   b a stock book?

Computers

Businesses are becoming increasingly aware of the benefits of computerised record keeping. All sorts of information, such as clients' details, appointments, stock records and sales figures can be stored on a disc. The information can be retrieved easily by a trained person. Some manufacturers produce software (programmes) specially for use in a salon.

If you use a computer you should copy recorded information on to a second disc to provide backup in case of loss or damage to the main disc.

Consultation

In order to achieve a beneficial treatment plan for an individual client it is essential that the therapist carries out a thorough consultation to establish a clear picture of the client's needs and constraints. This can prove to be a lengthy process for the trainee therapist but with time and practice the process will become easier and quicker.

There are many reasons why a client books an appointment for a particular treatment:

* They have heard about its benefits from friends

95

- They have read about or seen advertisements in magazines or local/national papers.
- It has been arranged by a relative or friend as a gift.
- They have, in their eyes, a problem, e.g. excess weight, poor skin condition, cellulite, stretch marks, tension in the muscles.
- They have a problem but don't have the confidence to book the type of treatment needed for this and so they have booked another type of treatment hoping the therapist will boost their confidence and recommend a suitable treatment plan for them.

When carrying out a consultation there are a number of things that the therapist needs to establish: medical details, personal details, body condition, skin analysis.

Medical details

Information regarding the client's past and present medical history should give the therapist clear indicators as to the possible underlying causes of the client's problems such as: the contraceptive pill causing an increase in appetite leading to weight gain; steroid medication for asthma causing weight gain; restricted mobility due to recent scar tissue causing poor muscle tone; previous acne causing skin-pitting-type scarring; childbirth causing poor abdominal muscle tone. Taking medical details also enables the therapist to identify possible contraindications to treatments.

Note. Specific contraindications to individual treatments are dealt with in each chapter.

Personal details

The therapist will take note of personal client details such as name, address and telephone numbers for their client data base. A data base can be used for a variety of things such as for marketing purposes, e.g. notifying customers of special offers and new product/equipment launches. They are also useful in case of emergencies, such as therapist illness, where an appointment needs to be altered or confirmed.

Taking personal and medical details during the consultation procedure enables the therapist to establish a professional rapport with the client, to put apprehensive clients at ease and to build up a clear picture of the individual client. Information on the client's lifestyle and occupation assist in analysing the client's constraints (time and finances) which have to be taken into consideration when organising a treatment plan for the client. This can also help the therapist in analysing the cause of the client's problem, e.g. a sales representative's job would generally involve a great deal of driving which could lead to tension in the trapezius muscle and kyphosis

A therapist would automatically consider the general health of their client as this can affect many different aspects such as skin condition, posture, etc. It is also useful to consider the client's intake of such things as alcohol, coffee and tea, particularly if the client suffers with cellulite or fluid retention. Tobacco can cause dehydration of the skin as well as generally being an unhealthy habit. Diet plays a large part in our health so this should be taken into consideration as well. A poor diet can affect many of the body functions and systems, e.g. insufficient water could lead to constipation which in turn can bring about poor skin condition.

Female clients may suffer with skin related problems such as 'breakouts' due to their menstrual cycle, or they may suffer with pre-menstrual syndrome which may affect their general well being and cause many problems such as dehydration of the skin due to stress. The menstrual cycle brings about many changes in the client's body due to the hormonal balance and it is very useful to establish the time of the month prior to treatment, e.g. pre-menstrual, post-menstrual or mid-cycle.

Exposure to ultra-violet radiation is also noted in the consultation process as this can effect the client's skin condition and the sensitivity of the skin.

POINTS TO NOTE ▷

- *A client who suffers with lower back ache in pre-menstrual cycle may benefit from a back massage for relaxation.*
- *Sunburn in the area of treatment is a contraindication.*
- *Exposure to ultra-violet radiation can cause dehydration and aging of the skin.*
- *A professional therapist will always consider the client as an individual and where needed recommend an alternative therapist for treatments that they are not qualified to offer. For example, if a client has superfluous hair due to hormonal change such as pregnancy, the therapist would recommend electrical epilation which may or may not be included in their clinical practice.*

Fig. 3.15 *Body condition*

Body condition

At the initial consultation for body treatments the therapist would establish the client's weight, height, frame size and body type, e.g. ectomorph, endomorph, mesomorph or combination. If the client was extremely sensitive about their weight at the initial consultation the therapist could offer a questionnaire with a number of weight variables to ascertain an approximate guide for organising a treatment plan.

Testing of the client's muscle tone is undertaken to establish any weak areas. The therapist would also note types of adipose tissue, e.g. cellulite, soft tissue and the area of the deposits along with any varicose veins or broken capillaries which may contraindicate treatment and the condition of the client's circulation, e.g. good, poor, fluid retention.

A thorough figure and posture analysis is carried out to highlight any problem areas and the client's reasons for treatment are recorded. All of these points will have assisted the therapist in establishing a total picture of the client's needs in order for them to develop a realistic treatment plan for the individual client.

Figure 3.16 shows an example of a trainee's consultation card for body treatments.

Medical details	Personal details
Name of doctor:	Name of client:
Present medication:	Address:
Past medication:	
Number of pregnancies:	Home tel.: Work tel.:
Ages of children:	Date of birth:
Operations: Hysterectomy ( ) Caesarean section ( )	Lifestyle:
Others	Occupation:
	Smoker (Y/N) Number per week:
Contraindications: Diabetes ( ) Epilepsy ( ) Pacemaker ( ) Heart condition ( ) Asthma ( ) Thrombosis/phlebitis ( ) Metal pins/plates ( ) Skin diseases/disorders ( ) Oedema ( ) Blood pressure (high/low) Recent scars (up to 12 months) ( ) Hepatitis/blood infections (up to 24 months) ( ) Cuts/bruises ( )	Drink (units per week): Alcohol ( ) Coffee ( ) Tea ( ) Diet: Digestion: General health (good/poor) Exposure to ultra-violet/skin condition:

Body condition
Height: Weight: Frame size (small/medium/large)
Body type (ectomorph/endomorph/mesomorph/combination)
Muscle tone (please use the following symbols: + good, = medium, − poor):
Biceps/triceps ( )   Abdominals ( )   Abductors ( )   Adductors ( )   Gluteals ( )   Other
Types of adipose deposit (hard/medium/soft/cellulite)
Areas of adipose deposit:
Areas of cellulite:
Varicose veins/broken capillaries: Circulation (good/poor/fluid retention)
Figure/posture analysis: Scoliosis ( )   Kyphosis ( )   Lordosis ( )   Other
Reason for treatment:

Treatment plan	
Recommended retail/home care advice:	Recommended salon treatments:
Eyes	
Face	
Neck	
Decollete	Recommended salon products:
Bust	Dietary/exercise advice:
Body	

Note. The reverse of this card can be used for recording a client's measurements when undertaking figure improvement programmes.
Indemnity: I confirm that to the best of my knowledge the answers that I have given are correct and that I have not withheld any information.
Signatures of: Client: Date:
Therapist: Date:

Fig. 3.16 *Example of a trainee's consultation card for body treatments*

POINTS TO NOTE ▷ *Before stress can be dealt with effectively the therapist must be able to recognise its symptoms.*

- **Physical symptoms of stress:** *tension headaches; indigestion; muscle tension; dry mouth and throat; tiredness; menstrual problems; diarrhoea/ frequent urination; constipation; clumsiness.*
- **Emotional symptoms of stress:** *rapid mood swings; lack of concentration; indecision; feeling tearful.*
- **Behavioural symptoms of stress:** *sleep problems; overeating or loss of appetite; withdrawal from friends and work colleagues; increase in smoking/ alcohol intake.*

Skin Analysis

Analysis of the client's skin condition and turgor (tone) will enable the therapist to evaluate their needs. On a consultation card used for training a list of the main muscles or areas affecting expression lines could be listed to assist the trainee in recalling the key areas to consider along with possible problems the client might experience, e.g. comedones, areas of flakiness, poor elasticity, acne rosacea. An area for the therapist to note additional comments such as if the client has used products like Retinoic A which could contraindicate them to treatments such as waxing, or to note previous treatments and products used. The reason for treatment needs to be established during the consultation procedure to ensure that the therapist can organise an effective treatment plan. Skin analysis can be studied in depth in A *Practical Guide to Beauty Therapy* by Janet Simms published by Stanley Thornes.

Figure 3.17 shows an example of a trainee's consultation card for facial treatments.

POINT TO NOTE ▷ *After six treatments it is recommended that a new consultation card is completed.*

POINT TO NOTE ▷ *Retinoic A is a topical skin care product developed in the 1960s to treat acne. It speeds up exfoliation by reducing the stratum corneum from 14 cells thick to 4. Following the interest in Retinoic A other types of acids have been examined and used to speed up skin exfoliation. (See Chapter 7).*

Treatment plan

The therapist is now able to recommend salon treatments, identify a suitable salon range of products and the appropriate retail products for

Medical details	Personal details
Name of doctor:	Name of client:
Present medication:	Address:
Past medication:	
Number of pregnancies:	Home tel.: Work tel.:
Ages of children:	Date of birth:
Operations: Hysterectomy ( ) Caesarean section ( )	Lifestyle:
Others	Occupation:
	Smoker (Y/N) Number per week:
Contraindications: Diabetes ( ) Epilepsy ( ) Pacemaker ( ) Heart condition ( ) Asthma ( ) Thrombosis/phlebitis ( ) Metal pins/plates ( ) Skin diseases/disorders ( ) Oedema ( ) Blood pressure (high/low) Recent scars (up to 12 months) ( ) Hepatitis/blood infections (up to 24 months) ( ) Cuts/bruises ( ) General health (good/poor)	Drink (units per week): Alcohol ( ) Coffee ( ) Tea ( ) Diet: Digestion: General health (good/poor) Exposure to ultra-violet/skin condition:

Skin analysis	
Muscle tone (please use the following symbols: + good, = medium, − poor):	
Decollete ( ) Neck ( ) Mandible ( ) Zygomaticus ( )	Orbicularis occuli ( )
Skin turgour (tone):	Areas of pigmentation:
Areas of broken capillaries:	Type of pigmentation/vein:
Skin texture:	
Oedema:	Collagen/elasticity:
Open pores:	Comedones (open/closed/micro)
Papules:	Pustules:
Moles:	Superfluous hair:
Area of flakiness:	Area of shininess:
Seborrhea:	Acne rosacea:
Acne vulgaris:	Dermatitis/eczema:
Psoriasis:	Skin tags:
Dehydration:	Scarring:
Skin type:	
Comments:	
Reason for treatment:	

Treatment plan	
Recommended retail/home care advice:	Recommended salon treatments:
Eyes	
Face	
Neck	
Decollete	Recommended salon products:
Bust	Dietary/exercise advice:
Body	

Indemnity: I confirm that to the best of my knowledge the answers that I have given are correct and that I have not withheld any information.

Signatures of: Client:	Date:
Therapist:	Date:

Fig. 3.17 *Example of a trainee's card for facial treatments*

Body treatment record card

Name of client:

Address: Home tel.:

                                            Work tel.:

	Date	Treatment, products and equipment	Therapist
Client's views on previous treatment			

Fig. 3.18 *Example of a body treatment record card*

the client and where applicable advise on complementary diet and exercise. (See Figs. 3.16 and 3.17.)

Figure 3.18 shows an example of body treatment record card.

POINTS TO NOTE ▷
- *A client is a potential client for all treatments and retail products that would benefit their skin and body condition, not just for the treatment they have booked.*
- *A client is paying for your professional advice and experience not just a treatment. It is their choice as to whether they adopt your recommendations, but they should always be offered.*

PROGRESS CHECK

1 Explain why you should consider the following when carrying out a client consultation:
   a personal details   **c** body condition
   b medical details   **d** skin analysis.

2 What two key areas form a treatment plan?

3 List three examples of:
   a physical symptoms of stress
   b emotional symptoms of stress
   c behavioural symptoms of stress.

4 State the information that should be recorded on a client record card.

— KEY TERMS —

You need to know what these words and phrases mean. Go back through the chapter to find out.

Viruses
Bacteria
Fungi
Animal parasites
Sterilisation
Autoclave
Sanitiser
Glass bead steriliser

Chemical methods of sterilisation
Disinfection
Antiseptics
Emergency first aid
AIDS
Hepatitis B
Reception

Receptionist
Dealing with clients, visitors and reception enquiries
Maintaining stock in the retail area
Consultation

4 Body massage

After working through this chapter you will be able to:

➤ explain the equipment required for massage

➤ describe how a welcoming environment can be created for a client having a body massage

➤ list the contraindications to massage

➤ name the main massage movements and their effects on the body

➤ describe the effects of massage

➤ perform an effective massage treatment for a range of clients including: male, female, apprehensive, for stress and relaxation, muscular aches and pains, weight loss, poor muscle tone and for a variety of times, e.g. one hour, half an hour

➤ identify different types of massage.

Introduction

Massage is much more than just manipulation of soft body tissue, it has deep psychological implications. Records show that ancient civilisations practised massage in varying forms before medicine was developed. Our earliest childhood memories of when we were injured are of adults insisting on 'rubbing' it better. Hippocrates, who is regarded as the father of modern medicine, made reference to the benefit of physicians being able to rub and knead.

So it can be seen that massage has firmly established itself as a therapeutic treatment and one which enjoys re-discovered popularity in our stress-laden times.

Over the last decade, massage therapy has expanded greatly. It is widely practised as a specialist field but is also offered by beauty therapists in salons, health farms, leisure centres, etc. One of the main benefits the therapist can offer the client is relaxation to release stress which can lead to aches and pains, postural problems, physical and emotional illness.

Every client from the high-powered executive to the busy houseperson will suffer at some time, if not for a large part of their life, with stress, whether through day-to-day problems encountered at work or in their social life or through a particular crisis. Stress can cause physical and emotional illness and therefore it is paramount that the therapist truly considers each client as an individual and views information gathered in the consultation to establish a full picture of that individual client.

A professional massage can be extremely exhausting both physically and emotionally for the therapist as they are not just laying on hands but giving of themselves. The majority of massage therapists ensure that they have booked sufficient time between each client to gather themselves and re-focus on the next person.

The consultation period spent with each client is highly important, it gives the therapist and client an opportunity to establish a professional bond and it enables the therapist to assess the individual clients' needs. On average the therapist would allow approximately thirty minutes at the first appointment and thereafter a minimum of five minutes should be taken prior to the massage to assess the client's reaction to the previous treatment and to establish their individual needs for this treatment.

Throughout the world, trainee therapists may learn different European massage routines depending on their individual tutor. When a trainee commences a massage programme the instructor will design an introductory massage routine which will encompass the classical massage movements and is generally designed to cover the whole of a female body and to last for one hour. This form of massage predominately affects the muscular and circulatory systems and is seen as a starting point to introduce the trainee to massage and develop their:

- manual dexterity and postural stance
- understanding of rate, rhythm, pressure and contact
- understanding of the classical massage movements and their benefits
- communication, organisation and management skills
- ability to analyse the individual's needs.

From the commencement of their training until the day they decide to stop practising and learning, the therapist will broaden their knowledge and technical skills by:

- observing various techniques by different instructors
- observing technical representatives from product companies
- observing fellow therapists in the industry
- watching demonstrations at beauty exhibitions
- receiving treatment from other therapists.
- reading text books on massage.

Once a trainee has learnt an introductory massage routine, mastering the correct posture, stance, rhythm, rate, pressure and client care, they will be encouraged to adapt their massage by drawing on their instructors' and other trainees' knowledge to suit the individual client's needs, e.g. male client massage is generally much firmer; clients suffering from stress in the upper back may prefer the time they have booked to be spent concentrating on this area.

Classification of massage movements and their effects on the body

Massage movements are generally divided into five main categories; effleurage, petrissage, tapotement, frictions and vibrations.

Effleurage

Effleurage can be defined as a stroking movement in the direction of venous return involving the pasage of the hand or part of the hand over the skin. The hand should be moulded to the area being treated and the fingers and thumbs should be kept together. It is.important that the pressure is constant and even throughout the movement. The pressure will vary depending on the area being treated; therefore effleurage movements can be subdivided into two forms.

Superficial stroking

As the name suggests, superficial stroking is performed using a very light pressure. The hand should be flexible and under perfect control so that the entire palmar surface is in contact with the area being.massaged.

Deep stroking

Deep stroking refers to the depth of pressure on the tissues rather than the use of force. Again the movement is performed using the entire palmar surface of the hand, but a greater depth of pressure is applied. The return stroke should be of a superficial nature, otherwise it may reverse some of the effects achieved, i.e. return of venous circulation and lymph.

Fig. 4.1 *Deep effleurage*

The beneficial effects of effleurage

* Aids venous circulation and return to the heart by the mechanical effect on the tissues.
* Aids lymphatic circulation by the mechanical effects on the tissues.
* Speeds the absorption of waste materials.
* Promotes relaxation by the reflex effect on the tissues.
* Enables the client to become accustomed to the therapist's hands.

Petrissage

Petrissage can be defined as pressure and/or relaxing of pressure. The movements consist of repeatedly grasping and releasing the tissues with one or both hands in a lifting, rolling or pressing fashion. Petrissage movements are often named according to the part of the hand used and include palmar kneading, palmar lifting, wringing, thumb kneading, finger kneading, skin rolling and picking up.

Fig. 4.2 *Petrissage*

Although the pressure is intermittent, care must be taken to avoid pinching the skin. This is prevented by gently relaxing the pressure as the bulk of the tissues diminshes.

The beneficial effects of petrissage

* Aids venous circulation.
* Increases lymphatic flow.
* Improves absorption of substances within the tissues.
* Loosens adherent tissues.
* Moves the tissues over bone.

Tapotement

Tapotement movements are sometimes defined as percussion-type movements which can be light tapping to beating movements applied in a brisk fashion. The whole hand or part of the hand can be used depending on the type of tapotement movement being given.

Tapotement movements include:

* Tapping – using fingertips only.
* Hacking – using ulnar border of the hands.
* Cupping – using fingers and palms of hands in a concave position.

Fig. 4.3 *Hacking*

Fig. 4.4 *Beating*

* Pounding – using the ulnar border of a lightly clenched fist.
* Beating – using lightly clenched fists palms down.

The beneficial effects of tapotement

* Very stimulating – causes erythema.
* Produces localised heat.
* Stimulates muscle fibres.
* Increases cellular activity.

Frictions

Frictions are normally performed with either the palms or the fingers or the thumbs. The superficial tissues are moved over the underlying structures keeping the hand in firm contact whilst performing small circular movements in a restricted area before gliding on to the next part. The movement is applied in a direction which produces tension on the tissues and has a loosening effect. Pressure should not be too firm otherwise bruising may occur.

The beneficial effects of frictions

* Loosens adherent tissues.
* Greatly increases localised circulation.
* Speeds cellular activity.

Vibrations

Vibrations are defined as rapid muscular contractions of the therapist's arms being transmitted through the fingers or palms to produce a highly stimulating, shaking-type movement. Vibrations are normally applied on areas overlying muscular motor points.

Fig. 4.5 *Frictions*

Fig. 4.6 *Light vibrations*

The beneficial effects of vibrations

⊛ Increases blood circulation.

⊛ Stimulates localised nerve endings.

Preparation for massage

Treatment area

Massage treatment areas vary in appearance depending on the environment in which they are found. Some salons have individual rooms for therapists to work in, designed to allow complete privacy for the client. Others screen the salon into a number of cubicles by using rails and curtains, like those you see in hospitals.

Equipment required for massage

Beauty couches

In order for the massage to be performed, a sturdy, comfortable treatment couch of the correct height for the individual therapist is needed. There are a wide variety of couches available for the therapist or salon owner to choose from.

A general purpose massage or treatment couch with an adjustable back support is available in standard heights. They can be purchased with a 'breathe hole' which can be removed when performing back and neck massage to allow the client to breathe easily. A face cushion can also be purchased and used where the couch does not have a breathe hole or when the therapist or client feels the need to use one to aid comfort during the treatment.

A multi-purpose couch is available in standard heights. It enables the therapist to convert the couch from a massage plinth to a couch suitable for facial treatments by lifting and lowering the client's legs for comfort and raising the back support.

Hydraulic couches have been developed over recent years to enhance the working life of the therapist as they can be adjusted to suit the height of the individual and/or the particular treatment they are performing. There are a variety of hydraulic couches available:

- The hydraulic massage couch (plinth) is a heavy-duty massage couch with a multi-positional back support which is raised by a foot-operated hydraulic pump. Such a couch would be beneficial in a massage treatment room which is used by a variety of therapists or for tall and small therapists working on their own who struggle with standard size couches.

- The hydraulic beauty bed (couch) is a heavy-duty beauty couch which can be manually adjusted for body treatments, facials or epilation and can be raised or lowered by a foot-operated hydraulic pump to suit the height of the individual therapist. This type of couch is extremely beneficial where a variety of treatments are offered and/or a number of therapists use the treatment area.

- The electrically operated hydraulic beauty bed (couch) is considered to be the present top-of-the-range hydraulic couch. It has all the advantages of the standard hydraulic beauty bed with the additional luxury of electronically moving some or all parts of the couch.

It is important to note that hydraulic couches:

- Protect therapists and employees from possible postural problems due to the use of couches of incorrect height and thus enables the therapist to perform a treatment more accurately.

- Enable a variety of therapists of differing heights to perform different treatments in the same treatment area.

Prior to the client's arrival the therapist or their assistant should ensure the couch is covered with clean linen, towels and/or blankets depending upon the salon policy or the client's preference. The couch may be covered with paper towels to maintain hygienic conditions, protect the linen and reduce laundry bills. Pillows or rolled towels should be available for client comfort throughout the treatment.

Couch steps
Couch steps are available to assist clients who are particularly small or who for medical reasons have difficulty getting onto the general purpose non-hydraulic couch. They should be used with care and always with the therapist in attendance.

Fig. 4.7 *Electrically operated beauty couch*

Beauty chairs (stools)

As part of some massage treatments, the therapist may need to sit to ensure they are able to apply the appropriate pressure and at the same time protect their own posture. Therefore there will be a need to ensure an operators chair or stool is in the treatment area. The important thing to note with this piece of furniture is that it has well oiled castors which allows the therapist to manoeuvre into different positions smoothly and prevents any unnecessary noise and that it should be adjusted correctly to suit the height of the therapist.

It is important to observe general safety in the treatment area by ensuring the chair or stool is safely stored to prevent any accidents.

Beauty trolleys

Most therapists use a sturdy trolley with easy-moving castors to hold the products and materials needed to perform a massage. Some holistic therapists may use a convenient surface such as a table rather than a traditional trolley to detract from the clinical aspect of massage.

Whatever surface is being used it is essential that it is cleaned and prepared with the necessary items before the client arrives and is suited for the purpose.

First impressions count, so it is essential that the therapist and treatment area are well prepared for each client.

ACTIVITY	Research the variety of massage equipment available. Draw up a chart detailing cost, durability and features of each piece of equipment.

The therapist

To establish a professional ethos, the therapist should take great care of his or her appearance and personal hygiene, particularly for massage treatments where they will be working in close contact with their clients.

They should always note the following:

* A high standard of personal hygiene should be observed at all times.
* Professional dress should be worn in the salon environment. It should be non-restrictive, clean and pressed.
* Items required to ensure personal hygiene can be maintained throughout the day should be kept in the therapist's locker, e.g. soap, towel, deodorant, a change of clothes, toothbrush and toothpaste.
* Hair should be clean and well groomed. Long hair should be styled to prevent it from falling into the client's or therapist's face.
* Comfortable, supportive, low-heeled, closed-in shoes should be worn to prevent poor posture and subsequent back problems.
* Nails should be short so that they do not disturb the flow of the massage or cause discomfort to the client and should be unvarnished for hygienic practice and in case of client allergy.
* Jewellery should be removed from the wrists and hands, along with dangling earrings or chains, again to ensure the flow of the massage and so as not to disturb the client's relaxation.
* A calm, relaxed, reassuring therapist is essential for a massage treatment.

Items required for massage

Essential items:

* Massage medium (lubricant).
* Tissues.
* Cotton-wool.
* Protection for the client's hair.
* Waste receptacle.

Optional items:

* Eau de cologne (for refreshing client's feet and/or removing oil/cream).
* Hot, damp towels (for removing excess oil/cream).
* Hot, dry towels (for therapeutic purposes).
* Footspray (for refreshing client's feet).

Massage mediums

Traditionally a variety of massage mediums have been used.

Oils

Oil still tends to be the most popular lubricant for body massage as it gives the therapist more slip. The oils selected by today's therapists generally have a base of vegetable or plant oils and may have other active ingredients added to create a particular effect on the body, e.g.

lemon (stimulating). Aromatherapy is a specialised massage treatment using essential oils for therapeutic purposes. This can be studied in depth by attending specialised training courses.

Modern therapists tend not to use mixtures high in mineral oil as these are generally considered to be comedogenic.

Creams

Cream is not a particularly popular medium for a full body massage, though it has been used in the past for spot areas of massage or because of a client's preference. Today you are far more likely to find creams being used as part of a particular manual body treatment for skin improvement, i.e. cellulite or stretch mark treatments.

Talcum powder

Talcum powder tends to be used as a lubricant when an electrotherapy treatment is carried out in conjunction with massage and the client or therapist do not want to use an oil or cream, e.g. during high frequency treatments. Talcum powder is popular with reflexologists as it gives 'slip' to the therapist's hands. It is often believed that greater depth can be achieved by using talcum powder as the massage medium.

In recent years product manufactures have greatly developed products available for salon massage treatments as well as for complimentary home care use. It is more popular to find a salon using one or two product companies' ranges rather than the old fashioned bulk products of the 1970/80s. One of the main reasons for this has been the huge technological advances of the 1990s, a great increase in the general public's awareness of product knowledge combined with their thirst for improved appearance and health. Therapists have also realised the professional and financial rewards which can be gained from retailing products such as body scrubs and lotions.

ACTIVITY	Research the different professional massage mediums available. Compare their ingredients and costs.

Creating a welcoming environment

As one of the main benefits of massage is relaxation, it is extremely important to create the right environment to enhance the massage treatment. This can be done in a number of ways.

Heating

As the client will be undressed during the massage, it is important to ensure they are kept comfortable:

* The room or treatment area may be heated to a higher than normal working temperature prior to the client's arrival and the temperature reduced as necessary throughout the treatment.

* Blankets can be used to wrap the client up snugly.
* Towels can be warmed over a radiator or in a tumble drier and placed on the couch for the client or over the area that has just been worked on, particularly on cold, damp, winter days.

GOOD PRACTICE ▷

* *Consideration should be given to the climate, e.g. in hot, humid countries the majority of clients like therapists to work in cool, air-conditioned rooms and to use cold (iced) towels on the areas that have been treated.*
* *Consideration should be given to the client's needs. Some people feel the cold more than others, e.g. in warm weather one client may not want to be wrapped up snugly in blankets and warm towels whereas another may prefer it.*

Ventilation

A well-ventilated treatment area is essential to prevent cross-infection of communicable diseases. It also ensures stagnant air, saturated with carbon dioxide due to exhalation from clients and therapists, is removed. A build up of stale air, containing heat, odours and carbon dioxide, can make the treatment room uninviting and the therapist lethargic which can affect the therapist's work.

Aroma

The treatment area needs to be inviting to the client and one of the ways the therapist can enhance this is by introducing aroma essence into the area. Qualified aromatherapists use essential oils for treatment and this obviously can create a pleasant smell in the treatment area. As no two clients are alike, the therapist must ensure that they know their clients' likes and dislikes in smells. The introduction of a smell the client dislikes will automatically prevent the client from relaxing and returning for further treatment.

Recently, a number of manufacturers have developed a small piece of equipment, a diffuser, which is used to introduce aromas into the atmosphere. Aromatherapy burners may also be used to further enhance the environment.

Fig. 4.8 *Aroma diffuser*

Colour

When planning a treatment area of a salon, the therapist should spend a great deal of time considering the decor (wall and floor coverings, towels, etc.) to ensure they create the right sort of environment for their clients. Generally therapists select warm colours, e.g. pinks, or relaxing colours, e.g. greens. The type of client plays a large role in selection of colour schemes, e.g. sports therapists may select white as a clinical colour and a beauty salon with mixed gender clients would generally avoid what are considered by some people to be feminine colours, e.g. pinks.

Colour used in a superficial form, such as in decor, towels and lighting, can contribute to a client's relaxation and should therefore be considered by the therapist when preparing the treatment area.

In recent years colour therapists have undertaken a great deal of research not only into the therapeutic effects of colour but into the use of light to heal (chromatherapy).

Lighting

Ideally the lighting of the treatment area for massage should be soft to induce relaxation. The use of strong bright lights can be very distracting to clients.

Sound

The therapist can perform the massage in a tranquil area and/or they may wish to compliment the treatment (with the client's agreement) with therapeutic music to aid relaxation. Some therapists retail taped music to clients who need to unwind and relax between treatments.

Health, safety, legislation and local bye-laws

Health and safety is of paramount importance and should be foremost in the therapist's mind. Therfore the therapist must be aware of certain legislative requirements in order to practise massage therapy. These are:

* The Health and Safety at Work Act 1974.
* The Office, Shops and Railway Premises Act 1963.
* Local government bye-laws relating to massage, e.g. Birmingham City Council Act 1990.
* Public Liability Insurance.
* Employers Liability Insurance.

(For further information on these legislative requirements and principles of good practice see Chapter 11.)

ACTIVITY | Through work experience, discuss with your colleagues how different salons have created a welcoming environment.

Massage consultation and assessment

The introduction to massage given in the earlier part of this chapter along with the chapter on consultation highlight the importance of performing a thorough consultation prior to the massage treatment to establish the individual client's needs, their views, preconceived ideas and to develop a professional relationship.

When training in massage therapy it is important to use a detailed consultation card which acts as a reminder to the trainee therapist to ensure they use all sources of information in order to establish a clear picture of each client. Once qualified, the therapist can purchase professional record cards or design their own for recording consultations and treatment depending upon their environment, e.g. salons offering a variety of treatments may use a multi-purpose record card whereas health centres specialising in alternative therapies may use a specialised record card.

In order to perform an effective consultation the therapist must know what the general effects of massage are along with the conditions which may prevent the client from having treatment.

The general effects of massage

- Improves blood circulation, therefore hastening the interchange of oxygen, nutrients, carbon dioxide and waste.
- Relieves muscular tension due to removal of waste.
- Increases lymphatic circulation, again hastening the removal of toxins.
- Causes hyperaemia which temporarily increases heat in the area of treatment.
- Helps to soften fatty tissue deposits depending on the movements used.
- Softens and nourishes the skin, depending on the medium chosen.
- Causes slight desquamation, thus improving the skin's texture.
- Skin tone and elasticity are improved.
- Stimulates or soothes the sensory nerve endings, depending on the massage movements used.
- Deeply relaxing – it gives the client a feeling of well-being.
- Helps to prevent stress-related disorders.

CONTRAINDICATIONS to massage

! Skin diseases.

! Infectious skin disorders.

! Vascular conditions – history of thrombosis, severe varicose veins.

! Heart disorders, high/low blood pressure (medical approval should be obtained before giving treatment in these cases).

! Unidentified swellings or lumps.

! Oedema.

! Raised body temperature.

114

! Burns/sunburn.

! Later stages of pregnancy (avoid abdominal massage once pregnancy is known).

POINTS TO NOTE ▷
- *If in doubt about the client's medical condition, refer the client tactfully to their medical practitioner without causing the client concern.*
- *Do not attempt to diagnose a medical condition.*
- *Some conditions do not prevent entire treatment, only treatment to specific areas or the omission of certain movements.*

Points to note in performing a consultation

On greeting the client, the therapist takes them through to the treatment area to carry out the consultation.

Details taken in the consultation should include:
- General details, e.g. the client's name, address and contact telephone number.
- Medical history details.
- General physical health details.
- Lifestyle details.
- Posture/figure analysis.
- Further salon treatments.
- Retail and home care advice.

(For further information on the reception of clients and client consultation see Chapter 2.)

Principles of good massage practice

1 Perform a detailed consultation so as to be able to devise the most appropriate form of massage to be given. The consultation is the basis to establish how best to treat the client's needs, i.e. type, duration and frequency of massage. The consultation is also needed to rule out contraindications.

2 Maintain good posture throughout massage. The therapist needs to ensure that throughout the massage routine he/she maintains correct postural stance for the movements and area of the body being treated to provide a benefical treatment for the client and to prevent fatigue of the therapist. When working on the body in a longitudinal direction use walk-standing and when working in a transverse direction use stride-standing (see Figs. 4.9 and 4.10).

3 Maintain an even rate and rhythm. Massage movements should be gentle, slow and rhythmical – with the exception of tapotement. The

Fig. 4.9 *Walk-standing – keeping the back straight, commence effleurage on client's foot, then glide up the leg rocking the body weight forward from heel to toe*

Fig. 4.10 *Stride-standing – knees bent, back straight*

acceptable rate of coverage is 18 cm (7 inches) per second and this should remain consistent throughout the massage to give the most beneficial effects.

4 Ensure hand flexibility. Manual massage treatment involves the use of the hands for maniupulation of body tissues. It is therefore essential that the therapist has complete control of his/her hands in order to mould them to the area being treated and provide the optimum treatment. When commencing training you should practise simple hand and wrist exercises to increase mobility and flexibility and use these exercises prior to a massage if the hands and arms are not suitably relaxed.

5 Adapt pressure according to the area being treated and the individual client's needs. The secret of a successful massage is to vary the pressure so as to be of maximum benefit to the client, but without being too heavy as to be uncomfortable or cause pain or bruising. Pressure should be increased or decreased gradually.

6 Always maintain contact with the client during the massage. When changing movements always keep a reassuring hand on the area to avoid breaking continuity of the sequence.

Preparation for treatment

⊛ Ensure the treatment room creates a welcoming environment.

⊛ Ensure the couch is protected appropriately.

⊛ The therapist should present him/herself professionally.

Fig. 4.11 *Hand and wrist exercise – loosely shaking hands and wrists*

Fig. 4.12 *Hand and wrist exercise – hands in prayer position, using alternate resistance push from side to side*

Fig. 4.13 *Hand and wrist exercise – rotate each finger and thumb individually in a circular fashion clockwise and anticlockwise*

Fig. 4.14 *Hand and wrist exercise – using ulnar borders of both hands, with relaxed fingers and wrists alternately flick the hands lightly onto a hard surface*

Massage treatment

- The client is greeted at reception and taken to changing area.
- Consultation is carried out to check for contraindications, to establish the client's needs and to explain the benefits of the treatment.
- The client may have a selected heat treatment to relax the muscles ready for massage and this treatment is carried out first.
- The client relaxes on couch, and using the selected massage medium the therapist performs a massage routine to benefit the individual client.
- The client is allowed time to relax and then offered a drink of mineral water. If the client wishes, the oil can be removed, either by the therapist or by showering. (Aromatherapy oil is generally left on the skin.)

PROGRESS CHECK

1 State the equipment needed to perform a body massage.
2 List six factors that will contribute towards a welcoming environment.
3 Give six contraindications to massage treatment and explain why each is a contraindication.
4 List the five classical types of massage movement and describe two benefits of each type.
5 State five specific effects of massage.

Introductory massage routine (for a female client)

The client should first be prepared by being asked to undress and put on a clean towelling robe. If possible, it is better to offer a heat treatment before commencing massage to relax the client and warm the body tissues. The heat treatment could be a steam bath, sauna, jacuzzi or even just a warm shower.

In the prepared treatment area, ask the client to remove their gown and get on to the couch lying face upwards (supine), assisting the client and providing couch steps where needed. Then cover the client in clean, warm towels.

POINT TO NOTE ▷ *The movements in the introductory massage routine (for a female client) are repeated a number of times to suit an individual client's needs.*

Front of leg massage

Preparation

a Remove the towel from the front of the leg area, keeping other parts of the body well covered for warmth
b Apply selected massage medium to the area by first warming it on your own hands and then applying it to the client's leg from foot to thigh following the effleurage pattern.
c Ensure your posture is good with a straight back.

118

Massage sequence

1 Effleurage to the whole leg

Place the entire palmar surface of both hands on the dorsal surface of the foot. With one hand leading, keep fingers and thumbs together and glide hands along the entire leg to the top of the thigh. Glide hands apart laterally, lightly returning to ankle.

(Main muscles affected: tibialis anterior, soleus, quadriceps, abductors, adductors.)

Fig. 4.15 *Effleurage to whole leg*

2 Deep wringing of the quadriceps

a Slide hands to interior aspect of the thigh and then with hands parallel, pick and lift the tissues and squeeze gently in a wringing action. Work the entire quadriceps area.

(Main muscles affected: quadriceps, abductors, adductors.)

Fig. 4.16 *Wringing to the quadriceps*

Fig. 4.17 *Effleurage to quadriceps area*

119

b Effleurage to quadriceps area.

3 Alternate palmar lifting of quadriceps

a Starting with hands on either side at the top of the thigh, use the entire palmar surface of both hands to gently compress the tissues against each other and lift from side to side. Keep repeating until the knee is reached and then slide the hands back up the leg.

(Main muscles affected: quadriceps, abductors, adductors.)

b Effleurage to quadriceps area.

4 Hacking to the quadriceps

a Using the ulnar border of both hands, briskly but lightly hack the quadriceps area in a rhythmical pattern.

(Main muscles affected: quadriceps, abductors, adductors.)

b Effleurage to quadriceps area.

Fig. 4.18 *Hacking to quadriceps*

Fig. 4.19 *Cupping to quadriceps*

5 Cupping to the quadriceps

a Holding the fingers and palms of hands in a concave position, briskly but lightly cup the quadriceps area.

(Main muscles affected: quadriceps, abductors, adductors.)

b Effleurage to quadriceps area.

6 Beating to quadriceps area

a Using lightly clenched fists, palms down, lightly beat the quadriceps area.

(Main muscles affected: quadriceps, abductors, adductors.)

b Effleurage to quadriceps.

Fig. 4.20 *Beating to quadriceps*

7 Thumb friction circles around patella

a Using the the thumb digits, gently perform friction circles around the patella.

Fig. 4.21 *Thumb friction circles around patella*

(Main muscles affected: tibialis anterior, soleus, quadriceps, abductors, adductors.)

b Effleurage whole leg.

8 Palmar kneading to the soleus

Using the thenar eminence of the hand push upwards along the soleus muscle towards the knee. Continue using the thenar eminence of the hand to apply friction circles in a clockwise movement, slowly working down towards the ankle.

(Main muscle affected: soleus.)

Fig. 4.22 *Palmar kneading to soleus*

9 Deep stroking around ankle malleolus
Using the digits of both hands gently stroke around the ankle malleolus.

Fig. 4.23 *Deep stroking around ankle malleolus*

10 Friction circles between the metatarsal bones
Using the thumbs of both hands apply friction circles between the metatarsal bones.

Fig. 4.24 *Friction circles between metatarsals*

122

11 Toe circles

Support the toe joints with one hand underneath the foot and the other on top. Circle hands in a clockwise then anticlockwise direction a number of times.

Fig. 4.25 *Toe circling*

12 Scissor friction on the sole of the foot

a Using the thumbs of both hands, friction in a scissor pattern down the sole of the foot returning with a deep push back.

b Effleurage to whole leg to finish.

Fig. 4.26 *Scissor friction on sole of foot*

Arm massage

Preparation

a Ask the client to gently lift her arm out of the towel covering.

b Apply the selected massage medium to the area using effleurage movements.

Massage sequence

1 Effleurage to the whole arm

Place the entire palmar surface of one hand on the client's wrist and

Fig. 4.27 *Effleurage to whole arm*

support with the other hand. Glide up the arm, around the deltoid, then lightly return.

(Main muscles affected: biceps, triceps, brachialis, deltoid.)

2 Deep stroking to the deltoids
Using the palmar surface of both hands, alternately effleurage around the deltoid area.

(Main muscle affected: deltoid.)

Fig. 4.28 *Deep stroking to deltoids*

3 Wringing and hacking to the biceps and triceps
  a Slide hands to biceps area and with both parallel, pick and lift the tissues and gently squeeze in a wringing action.
  b Effleurage area.
  c Using the ulnar border of both hands, briskly but lightly hack the area in a rhythmical pattern.
  d Effleurage area.

124

Fig. 4.29 *Hacking to biceps*

e Gently rest the client's arm in a crooked position at the side of her head (a towel support may be used under the wrist) and repeat wringing, effleurage and hacking movements to triceps area.

f Return the client's arm to its previous postion and effleurage the top of the arm.

(Main muscles affected: biceps, triceps.)

Fig. 4.30 *Wringing to triceps*

4 Effleurage to lower arm
Using entire palmar surface of hand, sroke the lower arm from wrist to elbow in an alternate fashion.

(Main muscle affected: brachialis.)

5 Friction circles

a Friction circle from wrist to elbow with a deep push back.

(Main muscle affected: brachialis.)

b Friction circle around wrist joint using both thumbs simultaneously.

Fig. 4.31 *Effleurage to lower arm*

Fig. 4.32 *Friction circles from wrist to elbow*

Fig. 4.33 *Friction circles around wrist*

c Friction circle between each metacarpal bone with a deep push back and continue this action down each finger to the tip.

d Effleurage hand and then turn over so the palm is uppermost.

126

Fig. 4.34 *Friction circles between metacarpals*

6 Friction circles to hand
Friction circles across the palm of the hands.

Fig. 4.35 *Friction circles to palm*

7 Passive exercise
Turn the client's hand back to a proline position and grasp the hand in your own, supporting the client's wrist with your other hand, then perform gentle, passive exercises clockwise, anticlockwise, forwards and backwards.

8 Effleurage whole arm to finish
(Main muscles affected: biceps, triceps, brachialis, deltoid.)

POINT TO NOTE ▷ *When performing the passive hand and wrist mobility excersises it is very important not to force the joint beyond its natural range.*

Chest massage

Preparation

a Gently lower the towel in the area to expose the upper chest area.

b Ensure the client's arms are tucked into the towel unless otherwise requested.

c Apply massage medium to the selected area using effleurage strokes.

Massage sequence

1 Effleurage to the chest

Place the entire palmar surface of both hands in the middle of the chest area, then gently work each hand outwards separately, sweeping around the deltoids, over the trapezius, and back over to the starting area.

(Main muscles affected: pectoralis major, deltoid, trapezius.)

Fig. 4.36 *Effleurage to chest*

2 Knuckling of the pectorals

Clench fists lightly and then knuckle across front of pectoral area.

(Main muscles affected: pectoralis major.)

Fig. 4.37 *Knuckling of the pectorals*

3 Friction circles to top of shoulder

Friction circle a number of times using both thumbs simultaneously in the bicipital groove of the humerus and shoulder area.

4 Stroking of deltoids

a Using the entire palmar surface of both hands, simultaneously stroke around the deltoid area in a clockwise direction and then in an anticlockwise direction.

(Main muscle affected: deltoid.)

b Effleurage to chest area.

128

Fig. 4.38 *Friction circles to shoulders*

Fig. 4.39 *Stroking of deltoids*

5 **Reinforced ironing**

Using double hand pressure, effleurage across the pectoral area in a figure of eight.

(Main muscles affected: pectoralis major, deltoid, trapezius.)

Fig. 4.40 *Reinforced ironing*

6 **Effleurage to the chest area to finish**

129

Abdominal massage

GOOD PRACTICE ▷
* *Avoid abdominal massage if the client has just eaten a heavy meal.*
* *Abdominal massage needs to be lighter than massage on other parts of the body.*
* *Advise the client the abdominal massage may stimulate bowel and/or bladder action.*
* *Clients who are menstruating may prefer this area to be left out of the sequence.*

CONTRAINDICATIONS   to abdominal massage

! Pregnancy.

! Diarrhoea.

! Within one hour of a heavy meal.

Preparation

a   Place a rolled towel or small pillow under the client's knees to relax the abdominal wall. Remove the towel in the abdominal area keeping other parts of the body well covered for warmth.

b   Apply the selected massage medium to the area by first warming it on your own hands and then applying it to the client's abdomen following the effleurage pattern.

c   Ensure that your posture is good, with a straight back and stand with your right thigh towards the couch but facing forwards as in walk-standing position.

Massage sequence

1   Effleurage to the abdomen

Place the entire palmar surface of both hands on the abdomen and keeping fingers together, glide hands down towards the symphysis pubis, then glide under to the upper lumber spine where hands should meet and then glide lightly back on to the front of the abdomen.

(Main muscles affected: rectus abdominis, external obliques, internal obliques.)

2   Deep stroking of the abdomen

Place the palmar surface of both hands on the middle of the abdomen and then stroke in a circular motion following the direction of the colon.

(Main muscle affected: rectus abdominis.)

3   Wringing of the external obliques

a Still standing adjacent to the couch with the hands parallel, pick and lift the tissues and squeeze gently in a wringing action.

b Glide both hands across the abdomen and repeat to the other side.

(Main muscles affected: external obliques.)

130

Fig. 4.41 *Effleurage to abdomen*

Fig. 4.42 *Deep stroking to abdomen*

Fig. 4.43 *Wringing to external obliques*

131

4 Skin rolling to the external obliques

a Still standing in the same position with hands parallel, slide down the obliques and then feed the tissues through your fingers and thumbs in a rolling motion.

Fig. 4.44 *Skin rolling to external obliques*

b Glide both hands across the abdomen and repeat to the other side.

(Main muscles affected: external obliques.)

5 Effleurage to the abdomen to finish

(Main muscles affected: rectus abdominis, external obliques, internal obliques.)

POINT TO NOTE ▷ *The number of massage repetitions should be appropriate to the individual client's needs.*

At this point in the massage routine you are now ready to ask the client to turn over so that she is lying prone on the couch. This needs to be done as quickly and discreetly as possible with the least disruption to the client. Lift the towels slightly and ask the client to gently turn over. Re-arrange the towels neatly.

Back of leg and buttock massage

Preparation

a Remove the towel from the back leg area exposing the leg and gluteal area, but keeping other parts of the body well covered for warmth.

b Place a small rolled towel under the client's ankle for support.

c Apply the selected massage medium to the area by first warming it on your own hands and then applying it to the client's leg from ankle to buttocks using effleurage movements.

d Ensure your posture is good with a straight back.

Massage sequence

1 Effleurage to the back of leg and buttock

Place the entire palmar surface of both hands on the Achilles tendon area of the ankle. With one hand leading, keep fingers and thumbs together and glide hands along the entire leg to the gluteal area, glide hands around the gluteal, lightly returning down to the ankle.

(Main muscles affected: soleus, gastrocnemius, hamstrings, gluteals, adductors, abductors.)

Fig. 4.45   *Effleurage to back of leg and buttock*

2 Deep wringing to the hamstrings and gluteals

a Slide hands to the interior aspect of the thigh and then with hands parallel, pick and lift the tissues and squeeze gently in a wringing action. Work the entire hamstring and gluteal areas.

b Effleurage to hamstrings and gluteals.

(Main muscles affected: hamstrings, gluteals, adductors, abductors.)

Fig. 4.46   *Deep wringing of hamstrings and gluteals*

133

3 Alternate palmar lifting of hamstrings

a Starting with hands on either side at the top of the thigh, use the entire palmar surface of both hands to gently compress the tissues against each other, lifting from side to side. Keep repeating until the back of the knee is reached and then slide back to repeat sequence.

b Effleurage to hamstrings area.

(Main muscles affected: hamstrings, adductors, abductors.)

Fig. 4.47   *Alternate palmar lifting of hamstrings*

4 Hacking to hamstrings and gluteals

a Using the ulnar border of both hands, briskly but lightly hack the hamstring and gluteal areas in a rhythmical pattern.

b Effleurage to hamstring and gluteal areas.

(Main muscles affected: hamstrings, gluteals, adductors, abductors.)

Fig. 4.48   *Hacking to hamstrings and gluteals*

5 Cupping to hamstrings and gluteals

a Holding the fingers and palms of the hands in a concave position, briskly but lightly cup the hamstrings area.

b Effleurage to hamstrings and gluteals.

(Main muscles affected: hamstrings, gluteals, adductors, abductors.)

Fig. 4.49 *Cupping to hamstrings and gluteals*

6 Beating to hamstrings and gluteals

a Using lightly clenched fists, palms down, lightly beat the hamstrings and gluteals.

b Effleurage to hamstings and gluteals.

(Main muscles affected: hamstrings, gluteals, adductors, abductors.)

Fig. 4.50 *Beating to hamstrings and gluteals*

7 Pounding to gluteals

a Using the ulnar border of lightly clenched fists gently pound the gluteal area.

(Main muscles affected: gluteals.)

b Effleurage to gluteal area.

c Effleurage to the entire leg.

Fig. 4.51 *Pounding to gluteals*

8 Deep wringing to gastrocnemius and soleus

a Slide hands to the interior aspect of the calf, and then with hands parallel, pick and lift the tissues and squeeze gently in a wringing action.

b Effleurage gastrocnemius and soleus.

(Main muscles affected: gastrocnemius, soleus.)

Fig. 4.52 *Deep wringing to gastrocnemius/soleus*

9 Alternate palmar lifting to gastrocnemius and soleus

a Starting with hands on either side at the top of the lower leg, use the entire palmar surface of both hands to gently compress the tissues against each other and lift from side to side. Keep repeating until reaching the ankle, then slide back to repeat sequence.

b Effleurage to gastrocnemius and soleus.

(Main muscles affected: gastrocnemius, soleus.)

Fig. 4.53   *Alternate palmar lifting to gastrocnemius/soleus*

10 Light hacking to gastrocnemius and soleus

a Using the ulnar border of both hands, briskly but lightly hack the gastrocnemius and soleus areas in a rhythmical pattern.

b Effleurage to gastrocnemius and soleus.

(Main muscles affected: gastrocnemius, soleus.)

Fig. 4.54   *Light hacking to gastrocnemius/soleus*

137

11 Light cupping to gastocnemius and soleus

a Holding the fingers and palms of the hands in a concave position, briskly, but lightly and gently, cup the gastrocnemius and soleus areas.

b Effleurage to gastrocnemius and soleus.

(Main muscles affected: gastrocnemius, soleus.)

Fig. 4.55 *Light cupping to gastrocnemius/soleus*

12 Digital stroking to calcaneal (Achilles) tendon

a Using all the digits of one hand, gently stoke the area. (The other hand can be placed on the calf for support)

Fig. 4.56 *Digital stroking to calcaneal tendon*

13 Effleurage the entire leg to finish

(Main muscles affected: soleus, gastrocnemius, hamstrings, gluteals, adductors, abductors.)

POINT TO NOTE   *On the lower leg area do not perform the beating movement as the muscles are more superficial.*

Back Massage

Preparation

a   Unless the couch has a breathe hole facility, place a support cushion, rolled towel or similar under the client's forehead to ensure that the neck is straight.

b   Remove towel from the back area keeping other parts of the body well covered for warmth.

c   Apply the selected massage medium to the area by first warming it on your own hands and then applying it to the client's back area.

d   Ensure that your posture is good with a straight back and stand with your right thigh towards the couch but facing forwards.

Massage sequence

1   Effleurage to the back area

Place the entire palmar surface of both hands either side of the spine in the lower lumbar region. Glide up the back area and over the deltoids firmly, then return back to the lumbar area with a light stroke.

(Main muscles affected: trapezius, deltoids, obliques, latissimus dorsi, serratus anterior.)

Fig. 4.57   *Effleurage to the back*

2 Wringing of the upper trapezius and deltoid

a Slide both hands to the right side of the client's back in the external oblique area. Then with both hands parallel pick and lift the tissues and gently squeeze in a wringing action. The pressure can be increased over the upper trapezius and deltoid area to suit the client.

b Effleurage to back.

(Main muscles affected: trapezius, deltoids, obliques, latissimus dorsi, serratus anterior.)

Fig. 4.58 *Wringing to the upper trapezius/deltoid*

3 Light hacking of the trapezius and deltoids

a Using the ulnar border of both hands, briskly but lightly hack the trapezius and deltoids in a rhythmical pattern.

(Main muscles affected: trapezius, deltoids, obliques, latissimus dorsi, serratus anterior.)

b Effleurage to back.

Fig. 4.59 *Light hacking of the trapezius and deltoids*

140

4 Light cupping of the trapezius and deltoids

a Holding the fingers and palms of the hands in a concave position, briskly but lightly cup the trapezius and deltoids.

b Effleurage to back.

(Main muscles affected: trapezius, deltoids, obliques, latissimus dorsi, serratus anterior.)

Fig. 4.60 *Light cupping of the trapezius and deltoids*

POINT TO NOTE ➤ *Do not apply any tapotement movements over the spine.*

USEFUL INFORMATION

Tapotement movements are often omitted from the back massage routine.

5 Friction circles along the erector spinae muscles

a Starting at the sacrum, place both thumbs either side of the spine. Working upwards gently, perform friction circles until reaching the seventh cervical vertebrae. Gently work into the area, then return with index and middle fingers down either side of the spine.

b Effleurage to back.

(Main muscle affected: erector spinae.)

Fig. 4.61 *Friction circles along errector spinae*

141

6 Deep wringing of the trapezius

a Slide the hands to the trapezius area and then with the hands parallel, pick and lift the tissues and squeeze gently in a wringing action.

b Effleurage to back.

(Main muscles affected: trapezius.)

Fig. 4.62 *Deep wringing of trapezius*

7 Friction circles across trapezius

Using the thumb digits, gently perform friction circles across the entire trapezius area working on any nodules of tension.

Fig. 4.63 *Friction circles across trapezius*

8 **Deep stroking of the trapezius**

a Place the palmar surface of both hands either side of the neck. Firmly stroke down either side of the spine to the thoracic region, then glide out across the scapulae and up and over the deltoids to the starting position.

b Effleurage to back.

(Main muscles affected: trapezius, deltoids, obliques, latissimus dorsi, serratus anterior.)

Fig. 4.64   *Deep stroking of the trapezius*

9 **Deep stroking of the spine to finish**

a Place the entire palmar surface of one hand in the cervical region and using alternate hands, gently stroke down towards the lumbar area.

b Repeat the action a number of times, getting progressively lighter to finish.

(Main muscle affected: erector spinae.)

This is the end of the basic massage sequence.

Fig. 4.65   *Deep stroking of the spine*

143

Adaptation of massage to suit the individual's requirements

Having mastered the basic principles of rate, rhythm and pressure for the introductory massage routine, a good therapist will develop their skills and knowledge to design a massage suitable for their client's needs.

It is extremely beneficial to take treatments from other therapists, attend short training courses, read trade journals and attend exhibitions, all of which will enable the therapist to enhance their own techniques.

There are many reasons why a client may request a massage, among some of the most popular are:

* Stress.
* Muscular aches and pains.
* Weight loss.
* Poor muscle tone.

Massage for stress and relaxation

The majority of people at some time in their lives will suffer with stress through pressure of everyday living, e.g. it is amazing how tense many drivers become particularly sitting in heavy traffic. Stress has many different physiological and psychological effects on the body: it is often responsible for causing tension in our muscles which if left untreated will eventually affect our posture and may even affect our general state of health. As one of the main benefits of massage is relaxation, it is extremely beneficial for most people provided they are not contra-indicated to the treatment.

There are many forms of massage available to clients, all of which will vary in time and price depending on the type of establishment the client visits and its location.

One hour body massage

The therapist can use the petrissage and effleurage movements from the introductory massage routine along with any other they have learnt from further study, demonstrations or from other therapists to devise an individual programme for their client. This may also include lymph drainage movements if the therapist feels they are appropriate to the client's needs. They will need to carry out a consultation and ensure there are no contraindications to the massage.

GOOD PRACTICE ▷ *Remember there may be contraindications on a particular area of the client's body which will not necessarily prevent massage to other areas.*

Therapists may choose to alter the order of treatment depending on their own and client's preferences, e.g. many holistic massage therapists commence on the client's back, spending a great deal of time here as this is an area prone to tension. They then move on to the backs, then fronts, of the legs and quite often may effleurage both legs at the same time. The arms and chest areas are next, followed by a face and scalp massage. Note that massage of the abdomen is often omitted.

GOOD PRACTICE ▷
- *Remember massage is a very personal, individualised treatment as no two people are alike. The therapist must ensure they prepare the treatment area and perform a massage to best enhance relaxation of the individual client.*
- *In European winters, therapists often use pre-heated duvets or heated under pads to assist the relaxation of the client. Warm, dry towels may also be applied to the area that has been treated to further induce relaxation and maintain the warmth generated in the tissues.*

Half hour body massage

The majority of health spas, as part of their package, offer a half hour massage and therefore the therapist must learn to adapt a one hour routine without making the client feel rushed. Rate and rhythm need to remain fairly constant and pressure altered to suit the client. Some clients prefer to have the time spent on certain areas rather than the whole body, e.g. legs, arms and back. Always establish during the consultation with the client their preferences and any areas of tension. New clients will look for the therapist's professional advice or quietly accept the treatment they are offered. It is far more rewarding for the therapist to discover problem areas which will enable them to give the client a more beneficial treatment rather than make small talk which can often become repetitive.

Back massage

Many salons' and spas' price lists will include a half hour back massage. This can prove to be a very popular treatment as a lot of people at some time in their life will suffer from tension in the shoulders and/or back. This can often be the first massage that clients experience. Over the years people have tended to feel inhibited about exposing their body without first knowing the salon and therapist. In many countries, whether through religion or culture, body treatments are not as popular. The therapist needs to establish a professional ethos that is reassuring to the client and embodies their culture.

During the consultation the therapist needs to establish any particular problems the client may have, e.g. tension in the lower back, along with their likes and dislikes in aromas, sound, colour, temperature and pressure. This will enable the therapist to ensure that the treatment room and product selection will assist more fully in relaxation of the client. The massage techniques selected will help relieve tension in the

┌ USEFUL INFORMATION ┐

In hot humid climates, such as the Far East, clients generally prefer darkened treatment rooms and cool room temperatures. Towels or cotton sheets are usually used rather than heavy duvets or blankets. Therapeutic music is very useful to cover the noise of air conditioning.

145

problem area and will include mainly effleurage and petrissage movements and in particular, deep thumb frictions to the trapezius and erector spinae muscles.

GOOD PRACTICE ▷ *Ensure the client is comfortable throughout the treatment. Consider:*
- *supports under the ankles, knees, chest and head when needed*
- *comfortable room temperature*
- *appropriate lighting*
- *suitable couch/client covering*
- *appropriate therapeutic music*
- *correct pressure.*

Apprehensive clients

Often clients attending for their first treatment are apprehensive and will tend to talk to overcome their fears. The therapist needs to be reassuring and encourage the client to relax to ensure maximum benefit is gained. The introduction of therapeutic music and essential oils either in the massage medium or in the aroma of the room may help.

It is important to establish the cause of the client's concern so that the therapist is conscious of their dilemma. Generally it can be assumed that the client is apprehensive as they do not understand fully what the treatment involves and/or they are nervous of exposing their body and feeling vulnerable. The therapist should bear this in mind by considering how she/he would feel semi-naked in unfamiliar surroundings with a total stranger who is fully dressed! The therapist should ensure they fully explain the treatment to the client and allow them time to get on to the couch and cover themselves before commencing.

GOOD PRACTICE ▷
- *Always state clearly which items of clothing the client should remove.*
- *Inform the client which way to lie on the couch.*
- *Always respect a client's privacy and when working on a female's back use a small hand towel to cover the side of their breasts.*

Massage for muscular aches and pains

The therapist must first ascertain whether there are any underlying medical conditions which would contraindicate the client from treatment.

Having carried out a thorough consultation and where necessary having gained approval from the client's GP (this should be a note that the

USEFUL INFORMATION

It is invaluable to take treatments with different therapists in different areas of your country, also when abroad, and to share these experiences with other therapists.

client has brought from their general practitioner) the client should be given a heat treatment, such as sauna, steam or infra-red heat lamp, to relax the muscles prior to the massage. The therapist may even decide to use the infra-red heat lamp during the massage to increase the heat within the tissues, thus aiding relaxation.

As muscular tension can cause aches and pains, the therapist should devote more time to particular problem areas using deep kneading and calming effleurage movements. The increase of warmth to the tissues brought about by the increase in blood and lymph circulation will assist in soothing the client's aches and pains.

Massage for weight loss

It is a popular misconception that massage alone can induce weight loss. Weight loss is brought about by diet and exercise. However if introduced as part of a planned treatment and home care programme alongside diet, exercise and electrical treatments, massage can prove to be extremely beneficial.

There are many reasons why a client may be overweight, e.g. it may be hereditary, as a result of over eating or lack of exercise. Whatever the reason the fact that the client has sought help indicates a determination to address the problem. Many people address the issue themselves or seek assistance through therapists or weight loss groups. The therapist must decide with the client the best plan of action to suit their individual needs and constraints such as time and finances available. They must also ensure that there are no underlying medical conditions such as hormone imbalance, e.g. an underactive thyroid gland can cause obesity.

Once a thorough consultation has been carried out and medical approval has been sought (where necessary), the therapist can use her/his knowledge and skills to devise a suitable treatment plan including diet, exercise, electrical treatments and a stimulating massage routine which should include petrissage (skin rolling, wringing and picking up) and tapotement movements (hacking, cupping, pounding and beating) on the areas of excess fat. It may prove beneficial to include manual treatments for stretch marks as often when people lose weight they tend to gain stretch marks. If the client suffers from cellulite the therapist could also include manual treatments for cellulite in the treatment programme (see Chapter 7).

Massage for poor muscle tone

The causes of poor muscle tone are many:

* natural ageing
* lack of exercise
* after rapid weight loss which may be caused through such things as illness or stress, or may be self induced.
* after pregnancy.

To tone poor muscles the therapist would need to recommend exercises to increase the strength of the muscles. These could be supported by salon electrical treatments for muscle tone and a stimulating massage routine incorporating mainly petrissage movements to increase the client's blood and lymph circulation. Once again the therapist could also offer manual treatments and home care products for stretch marks. (See Chapter 7.)

GOOD PRACTICE ▷
- *Carry out a thorough consultation.*
- *Check for contraindications.*
- *If needed, seek medical advice.*
- *Ascertain the client's needs.*
- *As part of a treatment plan, consider the client's financial and time constraints.*
- *Prepare the treatment area and client to induce relaxation.*
- *Devise an individual routine with movements suitable for the aims of the massage.*

Massage for men

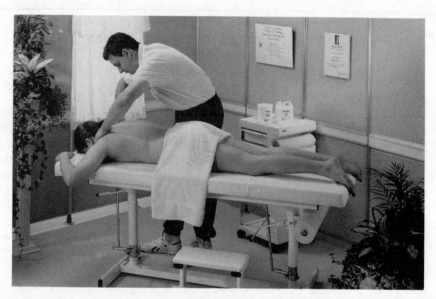

Fig. 4.66

POINT TO NOTE ▷ *Massage therapists (male and female) may treat members of the opposite sex, particularly if they work in a health spa, and must therefore:*
- *respect their clients' privacy by allowing clients time to undress and cover themselves*
- *adapt movements and pressure accordingly.*

Generally speaking males have more muscle bulk than females, course the female client is a body builder. As the muscles are and firmer, there is a tendency for males to have less subcut/ (fatty) tissue. The massage movements need to be performec. greater depth of pressure on men than on women. The type of movements used will obviously depend on the client's reason for treatment but would usually include petrissage (kneading, wringing and picking up), tapotement (hacking, cupping and pounding) and deep effleurage movements. If the massage is for relaxation then the tapotement movements would be omitted. As men usually have much more body hair than women it is important to ensure that the massage medium selected gives enough slip for ease of movement. Generally male massage does not include working on the inner thighs, abdomen or gluteal areas.

GOOD PRACTICE ▷ *Suggestions for after/home care and further salon treatments following a massage:*

- ⊛ *Allow a minimum of five minutes relaxation time after the massage.*
- ⊛ *Health spas often have separate relaxation rooms with reclining chairs, therapeutic music, subdued lighting and aromatherapy burners.*
- ⊛ *Advise the client to avoid strenuous activities for a few hours.*
- ⊛ *Recommend the client drinks plenty of water, particularly if essential oils have been used in the massage medium.*
- ⊛ *Having performed the massage and noted the individual client's needs, e.g. dry skin, stretch marks, cellulite, tactfully recommend a suitable treatment plan to include salon treatments and home care products considering the client's financial and time constraints.*

ACTIVITY

Select a client, perform a detailed consultation, devise an appropriate massage routine and justify your choice of movements.

Types of massage

Aroma massage

Aroma massage is generally for relaxation and uses ready-blended essential oils as the massage medium. It has become increasingly popular over the last few years and is practised by many beauty therapists. The massage routine incorporates mainly effleurage and petrissage type movements and is often enhanced by the use of therapeutic music.

The oils used in aroma massage are generally in a diluted concentration compared to those used by a qualified aromatherapist.

GOOD PRACTICE ▷ *Ready-blended aroma oils should only be used by qualified massage therapists.*

Aromatherapy

This type of massage is a specialist treatment which should only be offered by qualified aromatherapists. It uses plant extracts (essential oils) blended with a carrier oil to form a therapeutic treatment medium to suit the individual client's needs. The massage itself is the method used to transport the essential oils into the client's body and generally consists of effleurage movements.

The last decade has seen a great advance in the recognition of complementary treatments such as aromatherapy. Some aromatherapists work in hospitals under the direction of medical staff and a number of local health authorities have nurses trained and qualified in aromatherapy.

POINTS TO NOTE ▷

- *Aromatherapy is a specialist treatment given by qualified aromatherapists.*
- *Essential oils should only be used by qualified aromatherapists.*

Deep tissue massage

Deep tissue massage is considered to be a method of connective tissue massage. It involves a stroking technique which is used to stimulate the release of histamine from what are known as mast cells found within connective tissue. It increases the circulation in the surrounding area, and may produce a generalised flushed appearance and an erythema.

Lymph drainage

This type of massage involves working on the lymphatic system. True lymph drainage massage incorporates superficial effleurage and petrissage movements. Its aims are to relieve congestion within the tissues and increase the drainage of lymph to the lymph nodes. Generally clients come for treatment for specific problem areas rather than having a whole body treatment.

Multi-type massage

Multi-type massage originated in the Far East where it has been practised for many hundreds of years. It involves two therapists working in unison on the one client. It has recently become a fairly popular at a number of international spas. It involves a great deal of training to ensure the therapists are emotionally in tune and that their rate, rhythm and pressure are equal.

Oriental massage

Oriental massage has its origins in the Far East. It has been practised for centuries and is growing in popularity throughout the western world. Oriental massage is pressure massage using any surface of the the body e.g. thumbs, hands, feet, elbows, etc. It can also include gentle stretching

150

and manipulation along with the 'laying on of hands' similar t/ in spiritual healing. The application of pressure is usually b/ the meridian lines which are used in acupuncture.

Shiatsu is the Japanese name for oriental massage (*shi* meaning finger and *atsu* pressure). The majority of far eastern countries, such as Thailand and Malaysia, have, over the years, developed their own versions of pressure massage.

One of the main differences in oriental and European massage is that the client does not undress, though the therapist and the client need to be dressed in non-restrictive clothing. The massage is performed with the client either sitting or lying on a low bed or a mattress on the floor. It is also quite common in far eastern countries to see holiday makers receiving oriental massage on the beach!

Sports massage

This type of massage has greatly increased in popularity over the last decade, particularly as more and more people are adopting various sports as part of their leisure activities. The sports person is aware of the benefits of sports massage, which include easing aches and pains, and relaxing the musculo-skeletal system or specific muscles or muscle groups. Through specialised training the massage therapist uses a variety of movements to treat the individual client problem, e.g. deep friction movements are often used to break down scar tissue and adhesions.

ACTIVITY

Perform four massage routines on a selection of clients (male and female), who display different bodily conditions and age ranges. Keep a record of the body conditions noted, age and gender of client, the choice of lubricant and the massage routine devised.

PROGRESS CHECK

1 Give three reasons why massage treatment may be adapted. Explain each reason.

2 How would you deal with an apprehensive client?

3 Name and briefly describe four different forms of massage treatment.

KEY TERMS

You need to know what these words and phrases mean. Go back through the chapter to find out.

Effleurage
Petrissage
Tapotement
Frictions
Vibrations
Preparation for massage
Massage mediums

Creating a welcoming environment
Massage consultation and assessment
Contraindications
Principles of good massage practice
Adaptation of massage
Types of massage

5 Elementary science

After working through this chapter you will be able to:
➤ list the different states of matter
➤ state the difference between compounds and elements
➤ outline the differences between mains and battery electricity
➤ describe the effects of an electric current
➤ give examples of different electric currents used in therapy treatments.

It is beneficial for the therapist to have an understanding of elementary science, particularly before studying electrical treatments. A whole book could be dedicated to this subject which many therapists find fascinating and may wish to study at greater depth. There are a variety of books and articles available for further research to assist in performing effective electrical treatment programmes.

Forms of matter

Matter is anything that occupies space and possesses mass.

All substances can exist in three different physical states:
◈ Solid.
◈ Liquid.
◈ Gas.

Solids have a definite shape and distinct boundaries, e.g. ice, hair. The particles in a solid are packed closely together and remain in a definite position.

Fig. 5.1 *Forms of matter*

USEFUL INFORMATION

As the molecules in gases are far apart, they can be forced closer together, i.e. they are easily compressed, whereas in liquids and solids the molecules are closely packed so there is little room to push them closer together, i.e. they are difficult to compress.

Liquids have a definite volume and take up the shape of their container. The particles in a liquid are closely packed but have a certain freedom to move around.

Gases take up both the shape and volume of their container. The particles in a gas have large spaces between them and move freely (this is why we can smell perfume vapour from a bottle across a room).

All matter is composed of minute particles. In solids these particles are in definite positions, they vibrate in position but do not move from one part of the solid to another. The state of a substance depends on the energy that the substance contains. The solid state has a minimum energy content. When a solid is heated the internal energy is increased and particles vibrate more vigorously until it melts to form a liquid.

The state of matter is affected by temperature and pressure, e.g. if a solid such as ice is placed in a hot temperature, it heats beyond its melting point and becomes a liquid. Water, when heated beyond its boiling point becomes steam, a gas. This *change of state* from liquid water to gaseous steam is utilised in the salon environment when the therapist uses a steam cabinet.

Fig. 5.2   *Changing states*

Fig. 5.3   *The three states of water: ice, water, steam*

POINT TO NOTE ▷ *Cosmetics are temperature tested to ensure that they remain in the same state of matter. This is important to note when purchasing products for use in extreme climates.*

Atoms

Matter is made up of small indivisible particles called *atoms*, which cannot be created or destroyed.

For a variety of reasons, atoms can be attracted to each other to form *molecules*. A molecule is defined as the smallest part of an element or compound that can exist alone. Under normal conditions, elements which are gases rarely exist as single atoms, the atoms join together in pairs to form molecules, e.g. nitrogen gas.

Nitrogen atom + Nitrogen atom = Nitrogen molecule

Atomic structure

An atom is a particle of matter with clouds of *electrons* (which can be considered as concentric rings or shells) revolving around a small, dense mass of *protons* and *neutrons*, which form the *nucleus* of the atom.

* Electrons have a negative electrical charge.
* Protons have a positive electrical charge.
* Neutrons have no electrical charge.

Fig. 5.4 *An atom*

In atoms the positive and negative charges are equal, as they contain equal amounts of electrons and protons, therefore making them neutral.

Electrons fill the shells around the nucleus in a systematic manner. The first shell holds 2 electrons, the second shell holds 8 electrons and the third holds 18.

Elements are held together by forces called bonds. The ease of making or breaking these bonds is referred to as *chemical reactivity*.

The ionic bond is formed by the complete transfer of one or more electrons from one atom to another resulting in the formation of charged particles called *ions*.

An ion is an atom or molecule which has gained or lost electrical charge. The addition of an electron makes the atom or molecule negatively charged, i.e. it has gained the negative charge of one electron, and is known as an *anion*. The atom or molecule losing an electron will become positively charged, i.e. it loses the negative charge of one electron, and is known as a *cation*.

When therapists apply electrical galvanic treatments and products they need to know the relevant electrical charge of the ion in the product in order to perform an effective treatment. (See Chapter 6.)

POINTS TO NOTE ▷
- *Anions are negatively charged ions.*
- *Cations are positively charged ions.*

Elements and compounds

An element may be defined as a substance which cannot, by any known chemical means, be split into two or more simpler substances.

Elements are made up of one type of atom which cannot be broken down any further, e.g atoms of carbon make an element, atoms of oxygen are also an element.

When elements combine chemically together, i.e. *react* with each other, they form a substance. This substance is known as a *compound*, e.g. sodium chloride (table salt) is a compound composed of sodium ions and chlorine ions.

A compound is a pure substance containing two or more elements chemically combined together. Sodium chloride, hydrogen peroxide, keratin, etc. are compounds. Compounds have a fixed composition and their appearance and properties are usually quite different from those of the elements composing them.

When heated, copper nitrate gives off a brown gas and oxygen and leaves a black, solid residue. This indicates that copper nitrate is composed of at least three simple substances. The black solid and the brown gas can be split further. The brown gas (nitrogen dioxide) can be made to yield nitrogen and oxygen. The black solid (copper oxide) can be made to yield copper and oxygen. Copper nitrate is made of copper, nitrogen and oxygen. Copper, oxygen and nitrogen are all elements.

USEFUL INFORMATION

Copper oxide and nitrogen dioxide are both compounds.

There are over a hundred elements, most of which are present in the Earth's crust either in a free state or combined with other elements in compounds.

POINTS TO NOTE ▷
- *The constituents of an element, i.e. atoms, cannot be split into anything smaller.*
- *A compound can only be split by chemical means into the two or more elements that form the compound.*
- *A molecule is the smallest part of an element or compound that can survive alone.*

Mixtures

Mixtures contain two or more substances which may be elements or compounds mechanically combined. The constituents of a mixture do not react chemically with each other. A large number of preparations used on the skin are mixtures, e.g. calamine lotion, mascara and cosmetic creams are mixtures of fatty materials and water. A mixture can be separated into its constituents by physical means.

PROGRESS CHECK

1 List the three states of matter.

2 What two factors can affect states of matter?

3 Describe the atomic structure.

4 State what is meant by the following:
   a element   b compound   c mixture.

Electricity

We use the phenomenon and power of electricity everyday for heating, lighting, washing, ironing, cooking, etc. We use it to look after our appearance (shavers, hair dryers, etc.) and for entertainment (television, video, radio, etc.), but how much do we know about it?

Electricity can be defined as the movement of electrons from atom to atom. The moving electrons create an electrical charge which can be classed as either *dynamic* or *static*.

POINTS TO NOTE ▷

- *Dynamic electricity is electricity created by either chemical reactions or magnetic fields.*

- *Static electricity is created by friction. A common example of static electricity is the rubbing of hair with a plastic comb or brush. The friction between the comb and the hair can causes electrons to move from the hair to the comb. The comb becomes negatively charged as it gains electrons and the hair becomes positively charged as it looses electrons. As the hair and comb have opposite electrical charges they are attracted to each other making the hair stand out from the head and reach towards the comb.*

- *Electric current is the term used to describe the movement of electrons flowing freely in the same direction through a conductor to an area deficient in electrons.*

- *Conductors allow electrons to move freely through them, e.g. metals.*

- *Insulators prevent the flow of electrons, e.g. plastic, wood, rubber.*

Electric circuits

An electric circuit can be defined as the path of an electric current linking the electrical appliance to the electricity supply. To create a circuit two ingredients are required:

* a device capable of supplying electricity, e.g. a battery or a generator (mains)
* a complete path of conducting materials in which electricity can flow.

A circuit is made mostly of metals, but sometimes water containing dissolved acids, alkalis or salts can form part of a circuit.

a An electrical circuit must be made from a complete path of conducting material

When the switch is open the circuit is *broken*. No current flows and the bulb does not light.

When the switch is closed the circuit is *made*. Current flows and the bulb lights.

b Switches – 'making' and 'breaking' a circuit

Fig. 5.5 *Electric circuits*

Electric current

Electric current is the name given to a flow of electricity; it tells us the number of electrons passing a fixed spot in the circuit each second. Electric current is measured in amps (A).

Electrical pressure

This is a measure of the ability of a battery or generator to drive the current around a circuit. Electrical pressure is measured in volts (V).

Electric power

This is a measurement of the power used to run a piece of electrical equipment. Electrical power is measured in watts (W).

Electric cells and batteries

An electrical cell consists of:

● a plate made of a reactive metal, e.g. zinc

● a plate made of an unreactive conductor, e.g. graphite, carbon

● a solution or paste, called the *electrolyte*, containing acid, alkali or salt.

A chemical reaction between the metal plates and the electrolyte produces electricity.

A battery consists of several cells joined together.

POINT TO NOTE ▷

● *For a current to flow you require a potential difference (p.d.), i.e. there must be an area lacking in electrons and one with an excess of electrons connected by a conductor in order for current to flow.*

● *The resistance of a conductor refers to its opposition to the flow of current. The unit of measurement used for resistance is the ohm (Ω).*

● *Ohm's law states that the current flowing through a metal conductor is directly proportional to the potential difference (p.d.) across the conductor provided that its temperature remains constant.*

$$\text{Resistance} \rightarrow R = \frac{V}{I}$$

Resistance → R (ohms), p.d. (volts) V, Current (amps) I

Fig. 5.6 *Ohm's law*

The differences between mains and battery electricity

1 Batteries need replacing or recharging.

2 Mains pressure, or voltage, is much higher than most batteries. In the United Kingdom the mains voltage is 240 volts.

3 Battery equipment is usually portable.

4 Battery circuits conventionally have the current flowing from the positive terminal to the negative terminal all the time. This flow of current is in *one direction only* and is known as *direct current* or DC. An example of the application of DC current in therapy treatments is galvanic treatment (see Chapter 6).

5 The mains circuit produces an *alternating current* or AC (sometimes referred to as sinusoidal current) by continually reversing the polarity (direction of flow) of the current. An example of the application of AC in therapy treatments is high frequency treatment (see Chapter 6).

USEFUL INFORMATION

Ohm's law states that the electrical current will double if the voltage doubles, providing that the temperature remains constant and the resistance of the circuit remains the same.

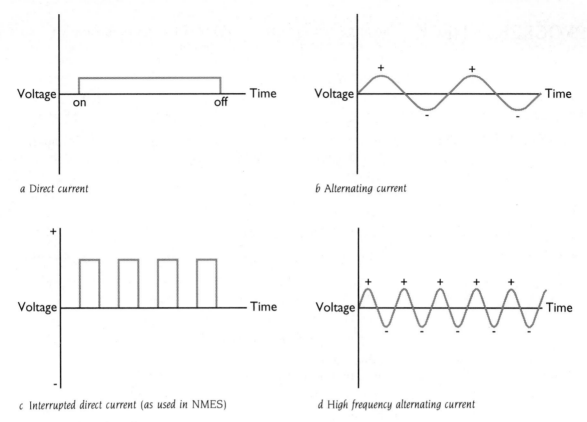

a Direct current

b Alternating current

c Interrupted direct current (as used in NMES)

d High frequency alternating current

Fig. 5.7 Electrical graphs

Earthing electrical appliances

Electrical appliances are earthed to protect the user from possible shock or electrocution.

Note. Appliances need not be earthed if:
- they have an all plastic body
- they are double insulated.

Fuses

There are two types of fuse:
- **Cartridge fuses.** These are placed in plugs to protect the cable of the appliance from overheating.
- **Wire fuse/circuit breaker.** These protect the wiring of the building from overheating.

In order to ensure the correct size of fuse and electrical cable diameter are selected for an electrical appliance, the current (measured in amps) must be calculated using the following equation:

Watts = Amps × Volts

or

$$\frac{\text{Watts}}{\text{Volts}} = \text{Amps}$$

PROGRESS CHECK If an appliance is rated at 1000 W (1 kW) and the supply is 240 V, what current is drawn by the appliance?

POINT TO NOTE ▷ To use any electrical appliance on the mains supply it has to be connected with a plug. It is important to note the colouring of the wires in a plug. In the UK the colours are:

● Brown = Live

● Blue = Neutral

● Green and yellow = Earth

The effects of an electric current

Heating effect

Heat is produced if you use:

● large currents

● thin wires

● resistance wires.

The heating effect can be used to good purpose in therapy, for example in the sauna stove and infra-red lamp element.

The chemical effect

The addition of salts, acids and alkalis (*electrolytes*) makes water a good conductor of electricity. An application of this effect in therapy treatments is the use of saline solution on the skin to enable conduction of an electric current, e.g. in neuro-muscular electrical stimulation.

If direct current supplies are used, chemical effects occur at the electrodes. An example of the application of this effect in therapy treatments is galvanic iontophoresis which describes the absorption of ions into the skin.

Magnetic effect

A current passing through a coil of wire (*solenoid*) causes the coil to behave as if it were a magnet, i.e. one end behaves like a north pole the other end like a south pole. If such a coil has a central iron core, the coil behaves as a much stronger magnet. The arrangement is called an *electromagnet*. This is a magnet which can be switched on or off as it only acts as a magnet when current is flowing in the coil.

An electromagnet supplied with alternating current will keep reversing its polarity. This is the basis on which an AC motor operates.

An example of the application of electromagnets in therapy treatments are mechanical massagers.

160

Electromagnetic waves

Wave motion

A wave motion is a disturbance travelling through a medium. Two sets of waves using the same medium can either reinforce or cancel each other out. This is known as *interference* and it can be used to prove that any type of electromagnetic radiation (i.e. heat, light, ultra-violet) consists of waves.

Wavelength and frequency

The *wavelength* is the distance between corresponding points on successive waves. It can be measured in metres (m), centimetres (cm), millimetres (mm), micrometers (μm) or nanometres (nm)

The *frequency* is the number of waves that pass any fixed point in a second. It is measured in hertz (Hz), kilohertz (KHz) or megahertz (MHz).

The higher the frequency, the shorter the wavelength.

POINTS TO NOTE ▷

* *The frequency of the mains electricity supply (AC) is 50 Hz.*

* A transformer *alters the voltage of an AC electricity supply but not the frequency.*

* A capacitor *charges with electricity and stores it until it is discharged. (A capacitor can be considered as acting as a spring, collecting power as it is compressed and then slowly releasing it as required.)*

* Rectifiers *change AC to DC as they allow the current to flow through them in one direction only. If a rectifier is used, then a capacitor is needed in the same circuit to smooth the current out.*

* The inductance of a coil *will oppose the flow of AC current. This type of coil is known as a choke.*

* A potentiometer *(often referred to as a 'pot') is used to control the intensity of currents. (The control knob on many beauty therapy appliances, e.g. galvanic, NMES, is a potentiometer.)*

* *The frequency of a high frequency machine will depend on the values of the capacitor and the coil.*

Costing of electricity

Electrical costs are based on the number of *units* used. The scientific name for a unit is a *kilowatt-hour*. To calculate the number of units the following equation is used:

$$\text{Units} = \frac{\text{Watts} \times \text{Hours}}{1000}$$

To calculate hours we transpose the formula thus:

$$\text{Hours} = \frac{1000 \times \text{Units}}{\text{Watts}}$$

Examples

1 How long will a 750 watt appliance operate for on 1 unit of electricity?

$$\text{Hours} = 1000 \times \frac{\text{Units}}{\text{Watts}}$$
$$= 1000 \times \frac{1}{750}$$
$$= 1\tfrac{1}{3} \text{ hours} = 1 \text{ hour } 20 \text{ minutes}$$

2 Calculate the cost of using a 3000 watt convection heater for 5 hours at a cost of 7.18p per unit.

$$\text{Units used} = \text{Watts} \times \frac{\text{Hours}}{1000}$$
$$= 3000 \times \frac{5}{1000}$$
$$= 15 \text{ units}$$

$$\text{Cost} = \text{Number of units used} \times \text{Cost per unit}$$
$$= 15 \times 7.18$$
$$= 107.7\text{p}$$

Fig. 5.8 *Inside of a dynatone machine*

ACTIVITY Research and compare the differences in the manufacturing of galvanic and high frequency machines.

PROGRESS CHECK

1 Give a definition of electricity.
2 Give an example of a:
   a conductor
   b insulator.
3 What is:
   a an anion
   b a cation.
4 State the two components required for the flow of electricity.
5 Explain what is meant by the following terms:
   a alternating current
   b direct current
   c volts
   d ohms.
6 What effect do the following have on an electric current:
   a a capacitor
   b a rectifier
   c a transformer?

┌─ KEY TERMS ──

You need to know what these words and phrases mean. Go back through the chapter to find out.

Solids	Mixtures	Electric cell
Liquids	Electricity	Earthing
Gases	Electrical circuits	Fuses
Atoms	Electric current	Effects of an electric current
Elements	Electric pressure	Electromagnetic waves
Compounds		

6 Electrical equipment for face and body treatments

After working through this chapter you will be able to:

➤ identify the different types of electrical treatment for the face and body

➤ list the contraindications to electrical treatments

➤ describe the effects of electrical treatments

➤ understand the preparation required for a variety of electrical treatments

➤ competently carry out a variety of electrical treatments for the face and body on clients.

Electrical equipment

A variety of equipment is manufactured internationally to meet the demands of the fast expanding beauty industry. The majority of companies produce a full range of electrical equipment, however some specialise in one area. Each company offers equipment at differing prices according to the development and design on offer and the back-up services available.

When selecting equipment, the therapist should carefully consider the treatments that can best be offered within the salon along with their available budget. Once these have been decided on it is wise to attend exhibitions, read trade journals and liaise through professional associations with other therapists before deciding which manufacturers items to purchase. If possible it is advisable to visit and view equipment showrooms to compare choice, range and availability of equipment.

There are a number of key questions that should be considered before any decisions are made:

* Is the therapist to offer salon-based or home visiting services?

* Where is the equipment to be used and stored?

* How much space is available for equipment presentation and storage?

* Would a multi-purpose unit be more beneficial if there is a shortage of storage space? (A multi-purpose unit could also be used as a point of sale for other treatments. However if it is the only piece of equipment, what happens when it breaks down or has to be serviced?)

* If the equipment has to be carried in and out of cupboards, is it light-weight?

* How are the electrodes stored – with the machine in a purpose-designed area or separately? How will this suit the salon environment?

* What is the durability of the equipment? How often will the equipment need servicing? Where will this occur – on or off site? How long will it take? What will it cost?

* What training is offered by the company? Is this included in the price? Where will it take place?

* What back-up services are offered by the company? Do they provide training manuals, telephone support? Do they charge for these services?

* What is the reputation of the company? Are they long standing? Do they attend the major international exhibitions? Are they active in more than one country?

* If purchasing from overseas, always check that equipment is compatible for use in the UK, e.g. check the wiring and voltage, repair and replacement of accessories, etc.

* Ensure items of equipment have been manufactured in accordance with current European directives (EU countries only).

Two of the major points that therapists do tend to consider when choosing electrotherapy equipment are the aesthetic appearance and the overall cost but these should not be the only points that are considered!

POINT TO NOTE ▷ *If the equipment is not under a guaranteed service warranty, take out a service contract with a local electrician who is familiar with beauty equipment. Ask the manufacturer or the local wholesaler if they can recommend one.*

Having purchased equipment, the therapist will want to use it to its maximum potential for the benefit of their clients. The services should be marketed well and full use of existing and passing clientele should be made including displaying information on the new services in the reception area, perhaps offering a discount for a course of treatments and an open evening to demonstrate the treatment and explain its effects.

Electrical treatments are generally given as a course. When used on the body, face, neck and décolleté a number of treatments are often combined together to gain the maximum benefit for the client. If the aim is for figure improvement, home care advice on diet and exercise should be given, and if it is to improve the skin condition, home care advice on the use of professional skin care products should also be given.

Care of electrical equipment

1 Hygiene is of the utmost importance so the machine and accessory items should be kept clean. (Check cleaning instructions before using solvents.)

2 Leads and plugs should be regularly checked to ensure there are no loose wires.

3 The equipment should be serviced regularly (portable appliance tested – PAT).

4 The therapist should ensure that all machines are maintained in good working order, kept in a safe place and that they are familiar with its operation.

Safety precautions to be observed when using electrical equipment

1 Ensure the correct care and maintenance has been given to the equipment. (Look for any signs of wear and tear, etc.)

2 Check the machine is placed on a sturdy trolley or where the equipment has its own built-in trolley, ensure the castors are firmly in place and that it is easily accessible for use. Never push trolleys or items on wheels, always pull.

3 Do not place water near or on top of the unit. Do not attempt to operate the machine with damp hands.

4 Make sure that there are no trailing leads that the client or other therapists (including yourself) could trip over.

5 Ensure that the machine is working correctly before applying to the client. Carry out simple self tests.

6 Ensure all accessory items, including products, are at hand before greeting the client.

7 Do not allow the client to touch any machine unless you specifically direct them to do so.

8 Test the equipment on yourself, explaining the procedure, its effects and sensation the client will experience.

9 Check for contraindications and where necessary test the client for skin sensitivity.

10 Before commencing the treatment, ensure all dials are at zero and that the machine is switched off.

Skin sensitivity test

When using electrical currents that pass through the body it is paramount that a skin sensitivity test is carried out to check the accuracy of the client's sensation in the area to be treated. It is usually performed by firstly testing the client's interpretation of different temperature extremes, by placing hot and cold water in glass containers, such as test tubes, and touching the area to be treated intermittently; then the client's sensation of touch is tested using a harsh and smooth surface, such as the pointed tip of an orange wood stick and the other end wrapped in cotton wool. Both these tests should be carried out with the client's view obstructed.

ACTIVITY

Research the number of equipment manufacturers available through your local wholesalers or main centres of electrotherapy supply. Compare their ranges, prices and back up services on offer.

Mechanical massagers

There are three types of mechanical massager available to the therapist, audio sonic massagers, percussion massagers and gyrators. These can be chosen according to the desired effects of treatment and the space available for storage within the salon.

Fig. 6.1 *Audio sonic equipment*

Fig. 6.2 *Ball massage head*

Fig. 6.3 *Plate massage head*

Audio sonic

An audio sonic massager is generally used to help relieve nodules of tension in the muscles. It is a small, hand-held vibrator that emits sound waves which produce a humming noise. These waves will penetrate 6 cm or more into the body's tissues and as the effects penetrate deep down it is ideal for sensitive skins. The action of the massager appears very gentle as it does not move up and down on the skin. It can only be used in small areas at a time due to its size.

The audio sonic is shaped like a small hammer. The external applicator head is directly attached to an internal electromagnetic coil or vibrator, whose action causes the applicator to move 'in and out' at frequencies in the audio spectrum, e.g. 30 Hz–20 000 Hz. The adjustable knob on the back or top of the unit is designed to restrict the distance that the applicator travels, thereby controlling the intensity of the massage application. A rocker on/off switch makes or breaks the electric circuit.

There are generally two massage head attachments sold with the unit:

- Ball massage head – used to intensify the actions of the vibrations in small areas.
- Plate massage head – used to evenly apply the vibrations over the largest possible area.

Percussion

The percussion type of mechanical massager is a small, hand-held unit which comes with a variety of massage heads, creating similar effects to manual percussion massage movements. A number of percussion vibrators have an intensity adjustment dial to enable the therapist to increase or decrease the vibration produced according to the depth of tissue being treated, they all have a main switch for turning the unit on or off. Percussion vibrators are generally used on the fine tissues of the face, neck and shoulders.

Different heads supplied are:

* Sponge head – used for gentle stimulation of the tissues.
* Spiky head – a rubber head used to create a more stimulating tapotement effect.

POINTS TO NOTE ▷

* *The intermittent alternating current causes the electromagnet of the vibrator to create an intermittent magnetic effect on the iron bar magnet within the unit which vibrates creating a tapping effect in the massage head attachments.*
* *The current alternates at 50 Hz releasing a tapping effect every half cycle (100 taps per second are emitted).*
* *If using audio sonic, a heat treatment such as sauna or steam bath may be given to relax the tissues prior to treatment.*

CONTRAINDICATIONS

to audio sonic and percussion

! Systemic conditions.

! Skin disorders/diseases.

! Bruised areas.

! Recent scar tissue.

! Highly vascular conditions.

! Varicose veins.

! Thrombosis or phlebitis.

! Over bony areas.

! Recent fractures.

Effects of audio sonic and percussion

* Increases blood circulation.
* Aids desquamation.
* Increases metabolism.
* Promotes relaxation through warming the tissues.

Reasons for using audio sonic

* Where use of other massagers such as percussion is contraindicated due to skin sensitivity.
* To help break down nodules of tension and relieve tightness in muscle areas, e.g. the trapezius.

168

⁕ For clients suffering with arthritis to create heat in the tissues which may help ease their aches and pains.

Reasons for using percussion

⁕ To stimulate blood circulation and sebaceous flow in dehydrated or dry skins.

⁕ To aid the texture of the skin through desquamation.

⁕ To produce warmth in the tissues to promote relaxation.

Preparation for audio sonic and percussion treatment

1 Observe general safety precautions for using electrical equipment.

2 The machine is placed on a stable trolley.

3 The machine is checked and tested to ensure it is working correctly.

4 The products required for treatment are selected and placed on the trolley.

Audio sonic and percussion treatment

1 Client is greeted at reception and escorted to treatment area.

2 Consultation is carried out to check for any contraindications and to explain the effects of the treatment.

3 Client removes their jewellery and is helped onto the couch.

4 The therapist ensures the client is warm and comfortable and prepared for treatment.

5 The appropriate massage head for the desired effects is selected and fitted firmly to the unit.

6 A suitable product medium is selected and applied to the area to be treated, e.g. talcum powder for oily skin and cream for dry.

Method

1 Check massage head is firmly attached.

2 Ensure that the unit is switched off and the mains lead is plugged in to the mains.

3 Machine is tested on the therapist in front of the client.

4 Massage heads are cleaned with appropriate disinfecting fluid.

5 The unit is switched on by turning the main switch (on/off).

6 The adjustment dial is altered as necessary.

7 Apply the massage head to the treatment area working in a methodical manner throughout the treatment either using circular movements or working in straight lines. Treatment time will vary between 5–15 minutes according to the area being treated and the effect required.

8 The unit is removed from the client's skin, the machine is switched off and where needed the massage head changed and the treatment routine completed.

GOOD PRACTICE ▷
- *Remember to avoid applying directly to bony areas such as the zygomatic arch or frontal bone when working on the face or vertebral column on the back.*
- *The therapist may apply the vibrator indirectly over more sensitive bony areas by placing the massage head on to their hand and working across the area to reduce the stimulation achieved.*

POINTS TO NOTE ▷
- *Avoid very bony areas.*
- *Ensure the tapping action is not too strong as this can lead to bruising.*
- *Do not use too close to the ears.*

9 The medium used is removed and further treatment may be given if appropriate, e.g. massage.

10 The client is helped from the couch, the record card completed, appropriate home care and further salon treatment advice is given, along with samples of the skin care products used if applicable, and their next appointment is confirmed.

11 The therapist tidies the treatment area and cleans the massage heads used with hot water and wipes them with disinfectant.

ACTIVITY

With a colleague perform on each other an audio sonic and percussion massage treatment. Discuss the physiological and psychological effects.

Gyrators

This is the most widely used mechanical massager and is commonly found in health spas and salons offering body treatments. It creates a much deeper massage effect within the tissues than the audio sonic and percussion vibrators. It is ideal for large muscular areas of the body and sometimes preferred by men with large muscle bulk to manual massage. There are a number of makes of electrical massage apparatus but the specific 'gyratory' action distinguishes this equipment.

The trademark $G5^{TM}$ is synonymous when describing gyratory massagers – the French manufacturer Monsieur Henri Cuiner created the very successful range of $G5^{TM}$ massagers over 30 years ago and the trademark derived from G for Gyratory and 5 from the number of accessory heads. Gyratory massagers are usually best used on a free-standing base with castors as this enables easier use and movement of the long flexible drive shaft, which runs from the body and motor of the unit, into which alternative massage heads can be attached.

A rotary electric motor inside the unit causes the crank and peg to fit into the massage head of the machine creating a gyratory (eccentric) movement.

USEFUL INFORMATION

An in-built air-cooling system is used to prevent the motor over-heating during constant use.

Fig. 6.4 *Gyratory massage*

Fig. 6.5 *Round and curved sponge massage heads*

There are a variety of massage head applicators available, the traditional ones tend to be made from rubber or polyurethane. The most commonly used or 'standard' accessory heads are:

* Round and curved sponge heads – used to create an effleurage effect. The curved head is used on curved areas of the body, e.g. arms, shoulders and legs. Used at the beginning and end of treatment. Increases blood circulation and produces hyperaemia in the area being treated. It also promotes relaxation.

* Single and double ball heads – used to create a deep petrissage effect on large muscle bulk, e.g. trapezius and gluteals.

Fig. 6.6 *Single and double ball massage heads*

* Egg box head (4 half domed head) – used to create a deep petrissage effect on fatty tissues, e.g. quadriceps and gluteals.

* Multi-pronged head – used to create a deep petrissage effect on fatty tissues.

* Spiky or brush heads – used to create stimulating tapotement effects.

Fig. 6.7 *'Egg box' massage head*

Fig. 6.8 *Multi-pronged massage head*

Fig. 6.9 *Brush massage head*

GOOD PRACTICE ▷

* *Plastic covers for the massage heads can be purchased which will help improve their life span and are better for hygienic practices. They also enable the therapist to work with oil.*

* *Some therapists use disposable plastic bags to cover the massage heads, which detracts less from the aesthetic 'feel' of the massage head and is ideal for hygienic use. It is important that a new cover is used for every client.*

POINT TO NOTE ▷

Fig. 6.10 *Water massage head*

- Water massage heads can also be purchased. Warm or cold water is placed inside the soft rubber head.
- There are a number of more specialist heads available for the traditional gyratory apparatus which are very useful to the experienced therapist.
- A Directional Stroking^{TM} adapter allows the applicator head to move in a simultaneous stroking and patting movement.
- A variable speed controller on a gyratory massager alters the massage effect and offers the therapist greater choice of application.

A hand-held unit is ideal for the therapist who offers a home visiting service or in a salon that has little storage space. This can operate on the same principles as the larger, heavy-duty, free-standing gyrator (but an electrical motor is housed directly in the body of the unit and no drive shaft is attached). Traditionally small, less powerful hand-held massagers are usually two handed and the massage heads are larger and often fit over the massage plate.

CONTRAINDICATIONS

to gyratory massage

- ! Skin disorders/diseases.
- ! Infected acne conditions.
- ! Bruised areas.
- ! Cuts and abrasions.
- ! Recent scar tissue.
- ! Sunburn.
- ! Sensitive and fine skin.
- ! Loose crepey skin.
- ! Oedema.
- ! Glandular swelling.
- ! Highly vascular conditions.
- ! Varicose veins.
- ! Thrombosis or phlebitis.
- ! Over bony areas.
- ! Very hairy areas.
- ! Over the abdomen during menstruation and pregnancy.
- ! Epilepsy.*
- ! Diabetes.*

* Only to be carried out with medical consent.

Effects of gyrators

- Increases blood circulation.
- Aids desquamation.
- Increases metabolism.
- Promotes relaxation through warming the tissues.
- Repeated electrotherapy pressure massage may help the more efficient dispersal of fatty deposits, particularly when the client is on a weight-reducing diet and exercise programme.

GOOD PRACTICE ▷ *A heat treatment such as sauna or steam may be given to relax the tissues prior to treatment. It is important that the area to be treated is sufficiently warmed before petrissage type massage is applied.*

Reasons for using gyrators

- To help break down nodules of tension and relieve tightness in muscle areas, e.g. the trapezius.
- For general relaxation.
- For improvement of poor circulation.
- To assist as part of a weight reduction programme for spot areas, e.g. quadriceps and gluteals.
- To assist in the improvement of the texture of dehydrated and dry skins.

Preparation for gyratory treatment

1 Observe general safety precautions for using electrical equipment.

2 The machine is placed on a stable trolley where necessary.

3 The machine is checked and tested by the therapist to ensure it is working correctly.

4 The products required for treatment are selected and placed on the trolley.

Gyratory treatment

1 Client is greeted at reception and escorted to treatment area.

2 Consultation is carried out to check for contraindications and to explain the effects of the treatment.

3 Client removes their jewellery and is helped onto the couch.

4 The therapist ensures the client is warm and comfortable.

5 The appropriate massage head to begin the treatment is selected and fitted correctly to the unit.

6 A suitable medium is selected and applied to the area to be treated if necessary, e.g. talcum powder.

POINT TO NOTE ▷ *When using massage heads with screw threads care should be taken not to cross thread.*

Method

1 Check massage head is correctly attached and will not loosen during treatment.

2 Ensure unit is switched off and mains lead is plugged in.

3 Machine is tested on the therapist in front of the client.

4 Clean massage heads are selected.

5 The unit is switched on by turning the main switch (on/off).

6 If the unit has a variable speed control this is adjusted accordingly.

7 Apply the massage head to the treatment area working in a methodical manner.

With the effleurage heads, follow the contours of the client's body and the direction of the venous return.

To create a kneading effect to the tissues the therapist selects a petrissage type head. This is applied in a circular motion allowing the kneading of the tissues. It is important to lift and support the client's tissues towards the head.

For a desquamating, stimulating effect the therapist selects a tapotement type head and works in circular movements supporting the client's tissues with their hand.

The treatment is always completed with the effleurage head.

The treatment time will vary according to the area being treated and the effect required, e.g. spot reduction or full body massage treatment. In some cases only a few massage heads will be selected, particularly if performing a full massage routine.

8 The medium used is removed (if appropriate) and further treatment may be given if indicated, e.g. neuro-muscular electrical stimulation.

9 The client is helped from the couch, the record card completed, appropriate home care advice given, e.g. diet and exercise, along with further salon treatment advice and the next appointment is confirmed.

10 The therapist tidies the treatment area and cleans the massage heads with hot water and detergent and then, according to the massage head used, wipes with a suitable disinfectant.

GOOD PRACTICE ▷
- *Ensure continuity is maintained whilst performing the treatment.*
- *Pressure should not be too heavy as bruising can occur.*
- *Support tissue areas as necessary during the treatment.*
- *Ensure the pressure from the head is kept flat and even to prevent damage.*
- *Massage heads must be stored only when thoroughly dry.*

POINTS TO NOTE ▷

● *As a safety precaution switch the unit on below the level of the couch in case the head is not firmly fitted and flies off.*

● *Care must be taken when selecting heads for the abdomen as there is no natural protection to the area from a bony superstructure, i.e. only the muscles and tissues of the abdomen itself.*

● *Mechanical massagers have been used by therapists for a long time, however in the past few years there has been a strong movement towards manual massage due to the psychological benefits gained from treatments that offer clients the warmth and understanding of the personal touch.*

ACTIVITY

Describe suitable gyratory massage treatment programmes for the following clients and conditions:

a 30 year old active male for relaxation

b 45 year old female office worker with hard fat deposits on thigh areas.

PROGRESS CHECK

1 Give six examples of questions that a therapist should consider before purchasing electrical equipment.

2 List the general safety precautions that should be observed when using electrical equipment.

3 Describe how a skin sensitivity test is carried out.

4 **a** What are the three types of mechanical massager available for salon use?

b Give three reasons for using each type of massager.

c List four common contraindications for the three types of mechanical massage.

5 Describe the preparation and treatment for one type of mechanical massage.

Vacuum suction massage

This treatment is used by therapists to assist in the movement of lymph fluid to the main lymph nodes, thus aiding the removal of waste products in the body. It also increases the efficiency of the circulatory system. It is generally given as part of a course of treatments and often combined with other treatments such as manual massage and dietary home care advice depending upon the area of the client being treated and the effect required. Treatment of the body using vacuum suction is often used for spot reduction in specific areas such as the thighs and buttocks rather than a full body treatment.

In order to perform this treatment effectively it is essential that the therapist has a knowledge and understanding of the lymphatic system (see Chapter 1).

Vacuum suction machines can be purchased for facial or body treatments. However the majority of manufactures produce mainly body or combined face and body units. These units generally consist of an electrically driven vacuum pump, a mains switch control, a gauge (which registers the amount of 'negative' or 'reduced' pressure produced) and a control dial for increasing or decreasing the amount of pressure required to treat the different tissues of the face and body. Accessory items to the unit are plastic tubing and an assortment of different sized ventouses or cups, which are generally made from Plexiglas or clear Perspex for the body and glass for the face. Some cups have a small hole in the side which the therapist places their finger over to maintain the pressure in the cup or to release the pressure when they want to. If there is no hole in the side of the cup the therapist has to release the pressure by gliding their finger under the cup. Some machines also have an outlet for blowing air out of the unit which can be attached via a nozzle to a bottle which will emit a fine spray. These can be used for a variety of preparations such as rose water for refreshing the client's skin.

POINT TO NOTE ▷ *The gauge on a vacuum suction machine registers the height of mercury on a sphygmomanometer. This was incorporated into the unit by manufacturers to meet the tuition requirements of some examining bodies who state the approximate measure that should be registered during use. The majority of therapists judge the intensity required by the percentage of tissue in the ventouse and how it actually feels to the client.*

Most vacuum suction machines available offer the therapist the single cup method of application. The multi-cup systems can be used for the body area enabling the therapist to work with a number of cups at the same time, thus reducing the treatment time. The method of application for this treatment is different but the effects achieved are the same. However these systems are not widely used in the salon environment.

The most widely used method of vacuum suction is referred to as the gliding cup method where by the therapist glides the chosen ventouse in a selected pattern and direction towards the nearest lymph nodes. Some units are designed to offer an additional pulsating action where intermittent pressure levels within the ventouse lift and drop the skin and body tissues as the therapist glides towards the lymph nodes. This method produces a gentle tapping effect on the skin producing stimulation in the area of treatment.

In body therapy treatments the therapist may select the gliding cup method for general lymph drainage, the pulsating gliding cup for further stimulation of the tissues along with lymph drainage or the static cup method for spot treatment in areas of fatty deposits, e.g. the thighs. The static method can be used to lift the tissues in a specific area and generally involves the multi-cup method of application, but can be performed by the therapist with a single cup outlet. The therapist selects

Fig. 6.11 *Pneumopulse vacuum massage equipment*

the appropriate size cups and applies to the treatment area ensuring the cups are moved around the area to prevent over stimulation and possible bruising. After treatment the gliding cup method is used to drain the lymph to the nearest node.

POINT TO NOTE ▷ *Vacuum suction massage simulates the manual cupping movement of massage.*

Vacuum applicators

- **Lymph drainage.** This ventouse can be used for most vacuum treatments. It has a flat, thin head and is useful for working in the fine facial expression lines.
- **Facial cups.** These vary in size and are generally used for general cleansing or lymph drainage.

---USEFUL INFORMATION---

As the tissue is released from the vacuum cup it falls and contracts, the contraction of the veins and lymph vessels forces their fluids on from the treated area.

Fig. 6.12 *Lymph drainage applicator*

Fig. 6.13 *Facial cups*

177

- **Comedone applicator.** These have a small, round opening which is used over the site of comedones, exerting even pressure on the surrounding tissues.
- **Body cups.** These vary in size depending on the amount of adipose tissue in the area being treated.

Fig. 6.14 *Comedone applicator*

Fig. 6.15 *Glass body cups*

POINT TO NOTE ▷ *The larger the diameter of the ventouse, the greater the reduced pressure will be at the same setting of depression.*

CONTRAINDICATIONS

to vacuum suction massage

- ❗ Skin diseases/disorders.
- ❗ Bruised areas.
- ❗ Cuts and abrasions.
- ❗ Varicose veins.
- ❗ Highly vascular conditions.
- ❗ Recent scar tissue.
- ❗ Sunburn.
- ❗ Sensitive or fine skin.
- ❗ Loose, crepey skin.
- ❗ Epilepsy.*
- ❗ Diabetes.*
- ❗ Any glandular swelling.
- ❗ Infected acne conditions.
- ❗ Bony areas.
- ❗ Very hairy areas.
- ❗ Thrombosis and phlebitis.
- ❗ Oedema.
- ❗ Heart conditions.*

* Only to be carried out with medical approval.

USEFUL INFORMATION

* The vacuum pump inside the unit is driven by an electric motor which produces suction in the ventouse by reducing the amount of air available thus causing the client's skin to be drawn up into the cup.
* The degree of reduced pressure produced by the vacuum pump can be increased or decreased according to the density of the client's body tissue by altering the intensity control allowing more or less air to leak which affects the amount of vacuum produced.

Effects of a vacuum suction massage treatment

* Increases blood circulation.
* Increases lymph circulation thus aiding removal of toxins and waste products.
* Aids desquamation.
* Improves general skin texture.
* Stimulates metabolism.
* Promotes cellular regeneration.
* Scar tissue may be softened.
* May help in the utilisation and movement of fatty cells when combined with diet and exercise.

Reasons for using vacuum suction treatment

* To assist in reducing cellulite.
* To assist in reducing areas of oedema (non systemic).
* For sluggish lymph circulation in specific areas, e.g. legs.
* To assist in a weight loss programme combined with diet, exercise and other salon treatments.
* To stimulate dry skin. The treatment time would be approximately 8–12 minutes.
* For deep cleansing very oily skins. The treatment time would be approximately 10–15 minutes.
* As a general skin cleanser on all but sensitive skin types. The treatment time for this would be approximately 5–8 minutes

General preparation for vacuum suction treatments

1 Ensure the unit is switched off and connect the mains lead.

2 The therapist selects the size ventouse required for the treatment area and attaches it to the plastic tubing which connects onto the outside of the unit.

POINT TO NOTE ▷ *The amount of reduced pressure being exerted on to the body tissues is registered on the vacuum gauge.*

GOOD PRACTICE ▷
* *When working on the delicate tissues of the face, the amount of reduced pressure exerted on the tissue will be a lot less than when working on the more dense body tissues.*
* *The ventouse should be inspected for cracks as these would affect the pressure.*
* *The therapist should ensure that the working ventouse surfaces are smooth and even so as not to damage the client's skin.*

Preparation for facial vacuum suction treatment

1 Observe general safety precautions for using electrical equipment.

2 The machine is placed on a stable trolley.

3 The machine is checked and tested by the therapist to ensure it is working correctly.

4 The products required for treatment are selected and placed on the trolley.

Facial vacuum suction treatment

1 Client is greeted at reception and escorted to treatment area.

2 Consultation is carried out to check for contraindications and to explain the effects of the treatment.

3 Client removes their jewellery which is kept safely by the therapist until the end of the treatment.

4 Client is helped onto the couch and their clothing and hair protected accordingly.

5 The therapist ensures the client is warm and comfortable.

6 The skin is cleansed with appropriate products.

7 A steam treatment may be given to soften the tissues.

8 A suitable product medium is selected and applied to the client's face and neck.

Method

1 A suitable ventouse is selected to suit the treatment area and the desired effects.

2 Check ventouse is correctly fitted.

3 Ensure mains lead is plugged in to mains supply and that all switches are off and all dials are at zero.

4 Machine is tested on the therapist in front of the client.

5 Check ventouse is re-cleaned with appropriate disinfecting fluid.

6 The unit is switched on by turning the main switch (on/off).

7 The intensity dial is adjusted to achieve the appropriate reduced pressure in the ventouse.

8 The cup is held in a perpendicular way to apply the ventouse to the skin. Remember not to draw more than 20% of the skin and tissues up into the cup.

9 Following the contours of the client's face and neck glide the cup slowly, to allow time for the effects of the treatment to be achieved, to the nearest lymph nodes.

10 The suction in the ventouse is released before the cup is removed from the skin by the therapist releasing their finger from the hole on the side of the cup or where there is no hole, by the therapist gliding their finger under the cup.

180

11 Following the pattern shown in Fig. 6.16, repeat the sequence to each area 4–8 times depending on the skin reaction.

12 If the desired effect of the treatment is to loosen stubborn comedones the appropriate cup is used in small circular movements over the problem areas which tend to be the nose, upper lip and chin.

13 The product medium is removed and either further treatment such as massage and/or a face mask may be given or the skin is toned and moisturised with appropriate products.

14 The client is helped from the couch, the record card completed, appropriate home care and further salon treatment advice is given along with samples of the skin care products used and the next appointment is confirmed.

15 The therapist tidies the treatment area and washes the cups and tubes used in hot water and detergent and then soaks them in an appropriate disinfectant.

USEFUL INFORMATION

In some far eastern countries it is common practice for therapists to perform the vacuum suction massage in conjunction with a steam treatment, this causes an erythema much more quickly due to the heat of the steam.

Fig. 6.16 *Direction of flow to the lymph nodes of the face neck and décolleté*

POINTS TO NOTE ▷

- *The loosening of blockages can be combined with the general cleansing treatment.*
- *When using the comedone applicator, cotton wool may be placed in the top of the ventouse to prevent waste matter entering the plastic tubing.*

ACTIVITY

Select two clients with differing skin conditions and carry out a minimum of six facial vacuum suction treatments. Describe the consultation, products selected, method of treatment, home care advice and evaluate the effectiveness of the programme.

Body vacuum suction treatment

1 Client is greeted at reception and escorted to treatment area.

2 Consultation is carried out to check for contraindications, to explain the effects of the treatment and decide on the desired effects required from the treatment.

3 Client changes, showers and may have a heat treatment to soften and/or another salon treatment, e.g. a mechanical massage.

4 Client is helped on to the couch.

5 The therapist ensures the client is warm and comfortable.

6 A suitable product medium is selected and applied to the treatment area.

Method

1 Suitable ventouse(s) are selected to suit the treatment area and the desired effects.

2 Check ventouse is correctly fitted.

3 Ensure mains lead is plugged in to mains supply and that all switches are off and all dials are at zero.

4 Machine is tested on the therapist in front of the client.

5 Check ventouse is re-cleaned with appropriate disinfecting fluid.

6 The unit is switched on by turning the main switch (on/off).

7 The mode of use is selected, e.g. pulsating method or static cup.

8 The intensity dial is adjusted to achieve the appropriate reduced pressure in the ventouse(s).

9 The cup is held in a perpendicular way to apply the ventouse to the skin. Remember not to draw more than 20% of the skin and tissues up into the cup.

10 a If using the gliding cup method the contours of the client's body are followed gliding the cup slowly (to allow time for the effects of the treatment to be achieved) to the nearest lymph nodes. The pattern shown in Fig. 6.17 indicates the movement sequence for working on the body with the gliding cup. The sequence is generally repeated to each area 4–8 times depending on the skin reaction.

b If using the spot treatment static or pulsating cup method, the appropriate size ventouse for the amount of adipose tissue is applied to the area. The suction in the ventouse is released before the cup is removed from the skin by the therapist releasing their finger from the hole on the side of the cup or where there is no hole, by the therapist gliding their finger under the cup and placed in another area.

Note. Trainee therapists sometimes combine the two methods of use, e.g. firstly using the gliding cup to loosen the tissues and stimulate the blood circulation prior to using the multi-cup spot treatment, which may help to loosen fatty deposits, before completing the treatment with the gliding cup to drain toxins and waste to the nearest lymph nodes.

11 The oil is removed and further treatment may be given, e.g. massage.

12 The client is helped from the couch, the record card completed, appropriate home care and further salon treatment advice is given and the next appointment is arranged.

13 The therapist tidies the treatment area and washes the cups and tubes used in hot water and detergent and then soaks them in a disinfectant.

Cervical nodes

Axillary node

Cubital node

Inguinal & sub-inguinal nodes

Popliteal node

Anterior   Posterior

Fig. 6.17   *Direction of flow to the lymph nodes of the body*

POINTS TO NOTE ▷
- *When applying the multi-cup static or pulsating method, a rocking action is used to roll the cups onto the skin at the same time to ensure the suction in the cups is equal.*
- *Care must be taken not to use too high a reduced pressure in the ventouse or to pull the cup of without releasing the pressure or to work in an area too long as all these can lead to dilated capillaries and bruising of the skin.*

GOOD PRACTICE ▷ *Drain to the lymph node, not over it.*

ACTIVITY

Plan a course of body vacuum suction treatments for a client with sluggish lymph circulation. Clearly outline the treatment objectives, describe the consultation, treatment methods and products to be used along with the client home care advice. Evaluate and justify your findings on the effectiveness of the programme.

Electrotherapy treatments

Therapists use the term electrotherapy to refer to electrical treatments where low currents are passed through the client's body for their therapeutic effects.

The three main electrotherapy treatments used by therapists are:

- High frequency.
- Neuro-muscular electrical stimulation (NMES), sometimes referred to as electrical muscular stimulation (EMS).
- Galvanic.

High frequency

The term high frequency traditionally applies to the high frequency apparatus used to stimulate blood flow and uses a rapidly alternating electrical current in the region of 100 000–250 000 hertz. It is a high voltage, but low current treatment. As the pulses of the current are short, they do not stimulate motor points to contract muscles – instead they pass directly into the skin via the electrode applicator at the point of contact producing warmth in the tissues which creates a heating effect. The therapist can apply high frequency in two ways depending upon the client's skin condition. Each method creates different effects on the

USEFUL INFORMATION

It is high current that kills, not high voltage. Remember 'volts jolt, current kills'.

Fig. 6.18 *Isis modular high frequency unit*

tissues:

* Direct method.
* Indirect method (often referred to as the Viennese massage).

POINT TO NOTE ▷ *High frequency is most popularly used on the face. However it can be used in the same way on the body.*

High frequency equipment may vary in general appearance as manufacturers develop equipment to appeal to therapists from an aesthetic and economical view but the basic operations of the equipment will be similar. There are generally two main control switches: the on/off switch and the intensity control. A mains lead connects the unit to the power supply. A flex leads from the unit to the handle which is used to house the glass electrodes. There are a variety of electrodes that the therapist can select to use depending upon the method of application and the area to be treated and the desired effects.

Electrodes

The glass electrodes have metal conducting caps (ends) which connect with the metal plate found in the handle allowing the current to flow from the machine to the electrode. The electrodes fit firmly into the holder but not tightly, otherwise the therapist would be unable to change electrodes.

* **Large head surface electrode (large mushroom).** This is used for facial and body work when using direct high frequency. It can also be used for 'sparking' treatments by using only on a side edge to intensify the current effected by lifting on and off the skin with small movements.

Fig. 6.19   *Large head surface electrode*

* **Small head surface electrode (small mushroom).** Used for direct high frequency. This electrode is useful for working on small, difficult areas such as the nose. It can also be used for sparking.

Fig. 6.20   *Small head surface electrode*

- **Roller electrode.** Used for face and body direct high frequency treatments. It rolls easily over the skin and can be used without gauze or a sliding medium.
- **Neck electrode.** Used for direct high frequency application to the neck area or other curved areas of the body, e.g. arms.
- **Sparking electrode.** Used for application of direct high frequency for sparking to specific areas and cauterising individual pores. Care should be taken to use a low current with this electrode.
- **Rake electrode.** Used for direct frequency to the scalp area.
- **Intensified saturator electrode.** This electrode is used for indirect high frequency and is known as a saturator. It usually contains a metal spiral running through the inside of the glass which intensifies the effect and ensures that only a low current is required to give maximum effect.

Fig. 6.21   Roller electrode

Fig. 6.22   Neck electrode

Fig. 6.23   Sparking electrode

Fig. 6.24   Rake electrode

Fig. 6.25   Intensified saturator electrode

POINTS TO NOTE

Within each electrode is sealed a small quantity of inert gas, usually argon. As the current flows through the gases a coloured glow is produced. The electrodes glow either blue–violet if they contain argon or red–orange if they contain neon.

CONTRAINDICATIONS

to high frequency

! Cuts or abrasions to the skin in the area to be treated.

! Skin diseases or disorders.

! Highly vascular conditions.

! Sensitive skin.

! Highly nervous clients.

! Excessive metal in the area of application, e.g. plates or fillings.

! Swellings in the area.

! Very hairy areas.

! Sinus blockages.

! Heart conditions.*

! Epilepsy and diabetes.*

! Circulatory conditions.*

! Pregnancy.*

! Asthmatics.*

* Only to be carried out with medical approval.

The indirect method

This method of applying the high frequency current involves creating a circuit of current which flows from the saturator to charge the client. The therapist massages the client, thus discharging the current from the client's face to the therapist's massaging fingers or hand.

Effects of indirect high frequency

* Increases circulation.
* Increases metabolism.
* Warms and relaxes the tissues.
* Improves the skin texture.
* Improves the moisture balance of the skin.
* Calms the sensory nerve endings.

Reasons for using indirect high frequency

* To improve dry or dehydrated skins.
* To improve tired skin.
* To help improve fine lines.
* To help relax the tissues.
* To help improve poor circulation.

Preparation for indirect high frequency treatment

1 Observe general safety precautions for using electrical equipment.

2 The machine is placed on a stable trolley.

3 The machine is checked and tested by the therapist to ensure it is working correctly.

4 The products required for treatment are selected and placed on the trolley.

Indirect high frequency treatment

1 Client is greeted at reception and escorted to treatment area.

2 Consultation is carried out to check for contraindications and to explain the effects of the treatment and skin sensitivity test is carried out.

3 Client removes their jewellery which is kept safely by the therapist until the end of the treatment.

4 Client is helped on to the couch and their clothing and hair protected accordingly.

5 The therapist ensures the client is warm and comfortable.

6 The skin is cleansed with the appropriate products.

7 A suitable product medium is selected and applied to the client's face and neck, e.g. massage or nourishing cream.

Method

1 Ensure mains lead is plugged in to mains supply and that all switches are off and all dials are at zero.

2 The therapist tests the machine in front of the client and reassures them where necessary about the buzzing noise it makes.

3 Talcum powder is applied to the client's hands to absorb any perspiration.

4 The saturator is wiped with disinfectant and placed firmly in the holder.

5 Depending upon the apparatus used the saturator is held firmly by the client at the free end, taking care not to hold over the point of electrode insertion into the handle. The handle can also usually be held by the client with their second hand but check the intended use with the manufacturer as in some cases this is not advised and the handle is supported by a towel.

6 The therapist places one hand in contact with the client's skin and begins to massage using small circular effleurage movements whilst with the other hand turning the intensity dial slowly, to suit the client's tolerance.

7 Place the other hand on the opposite side of the client's face and without losing contact, massage using both hands. The therapist should feel warmth in their fingers.

8 The treatment time will vary between 8–20 minutes depending upon the client's skin condition.

9 At the end of the treatment the therapist keeps one hand in contact whilst using the other to turn the intensity dial to zero before switching off the machine.

10 The cream is removed and either further treatment such as a face mask may be given or the skin is toned and moisturised with appropriate products.

11 The client is helped from the couch, the record card completed, appropriate home care and further salon treatment advice is given along with samples of the skin care products used and the client's next appointment is confirmed.

12 The therapist tidies the treatment area and cleans the electrode used by carefully wiping with hot water and then disinfectant. Special care must be taken not to wet the metal end connector of the saturator. All electrodes should be dry before being stored for later use.

POINTS TO NOTE ▷
- *The intensity dial may need to be reduced when progressing to areas of finer skin, e.g. the forehead.*
- *The intensity of the current in the tissues will be increased when lifting one hand off the skin during the massage.*
- *Tapotement movements such as tapping will intensify the current in the area being treated.*
- *In the past, talcum powder was used as a medium to create a stimulating effect, but its drying effects are not beneficial for a dry or dehydrated skin.*

GOOD PRACTICE ▷
- *Care should be taken when working around the hairline as sensation will usually intensify because hair is a conductor of electricity.*
- *Contact must not be broken. If the circuit is completely broken and then remade without turning the intensity dial to zero, the client may feel a stronger tingling sensation which may make them apprehensive of further treatment. However if the therapist wishes to intentionally create a stimulating effect on the skin they can slowly lift the fingers slightly off the skin and return them.*
- *Rings must not be worn by the client on the hand that holds the saturator (and preferably not at all).*
- *Care must be taken to ensure any belts with metal buckles are kept away from the saturator or removed.*
- *The client or therapist must not touch any metal conducting material whilst the indirect high frequency treatment is in progress, e.g. couch, trolley, etc.*

ACTIVITY

Research the variety of portable high frequency units suitable for use by a home visiting therapist. List the company names, cost, features of the equipment and back-up service. State and justify which unit you would recommend for purchase.

Direct high frequency

This method of application of the high frequency current uses glass electrodes which are placed in direct contact with the client's skin. The current is dispersed at the point of contact with the client and as the effects are concentrated around the electrode, they are superficial.

Effects of direct high frequency

* Increases metabolism.
* Warms and relaxes the tissues under the electrode.
* Improves the skin texture.
* Improves the moisture balance of the skin.
* Calms the sensory nerve endings.
* Produces ozone which has an anti-bacterial, germicidal effect on the surface of the skin. This effect can be intensified with sparking.

Reasons for using direct high frequency

* To improve the condition of seborrhoeic or oily skins.
* To improve the condition of oily areas, e.g. T zone, blemished skin on any area of the body.
* To aid the healing of pustule prone skins by using sparking on the skin
* To destroy bacteria through the creation of ozone through sparking.
* To stimulate secretion in a dry skin by treating the skin for a few minutes, e.g. 3–4 minutes.

Preparation for direct high frequency treatment

1 Observe general safety precautions for using electrical equipment.

2 The machine is placed on a stable trolley.

3 The machine is checked and tested by the therapist to ensure it is working correctly.

4 The products required for treatment are selected and placed on the trolley.

Direct high frequency treatment

1 Client is greeted at reception and escorted to treatment area.

2 Consultation is carried out to check for contraindications and to explain the effects of the treatment.

3 Client removes their jewellery which is kept safely by the therapist until the end of the treatment.

4 Client is helped onto the couch and their clothing and hair protected accordingly.

5 The therapist ensures the client is warm and comfortable.

6 The skin is cleansed with the appropriate products.

7 A suitable medium is selected and applied to the client's face and neck, e.g. oxygenating cream and gauze.

USEFUL INFORMATION

The application of the direct high frequency electrode creates warmth on the skin and converts the stable oxygen molecules in the oxygenating cream to unstable ozone molecules (which have a germicidal effect).

Method

1 Ensure mains lead is plugged into mains supply and that all switches are off and all dials are at zero.

2 The therapist tests the machine in front of the client and reassures them where necessary about the buzzing noise it makes.

3 The selected electrodes are wiped with disinfectant and stored safely for use.

4 The electrode is placed firmly in the holder.

5 The therapist either places the electrode in contact with the client's skin and moves it around using small circular movements whilst turning the mains control switch on and the intensity dial up to suit the client's tolerance, or places their finger in contact with the electrode before turning the machine on then the intensity dial up and placing both finger and electrode in contact with the client's skin before removing the finger.

6 The treatment time will vary depending upon the client's skin condition, e.g. oily skin 8–15 minutes, dehydrated skin 3–4 minutes.

7 At the end of the treatment, or between changing electrodes, the therapist must keep the electrode in contact with the client's skin whilst turning the intensity dial to zero and switching the machine off before removing the electrode from the skin, or place their finger on the electrode before lifting it off the client's skin and turning the intensity dial to zero and switching the machine off. Some units have a secondary on/off switch directly on the handle to assist with an easier change over of electrodes, etc.

Note. When sparking to create a germicidal effect which may destroy bacteria, the electrode is lifted off the skin. The distance created between the electrode and the skin should only be a few millimetres, causing the current to 'jump' from the electrode to the client's skin thus creating a spark which in turn produces ultra-violet rays which destroy bacteria. The germicidal effect is created by the ionisation of the oxygen in the air which creates ozone. Controlled quantities of ozone help promote the healing of pustules and papules. Pores are constricted when the sparks stimulate the skins nerve endings.

8 The selected medium is removed and either further treatment such as a face mask may be given or the skin is toned and moisturised with appropriate products.

9 The client is helped from the couch, the record card completed, appropriate home care and further salon treatment advice is given along with samples of the skin care products used and the client's next appointment is confirmed.

10 The therapist tidies the treatment area and cleans the electrodes used by carefully wiping with hot water and then disinfectant. Special care must be taken not to wet the metal end connector of the saturator. The electrodes are stored dry for later use.

USEFUL INFORMATION

* *To produce a high frequency current the equipment requires a capacitor and an inductor of a special type to increase the output voltage.*
* *Older style circuits used a spark gap inductor called a Tesla coil.*
* *The special transformer contained in the handle of the machine (which holds the electrodes selected for treatment) is known as the oudin coil or resonator.*
* *The actual flow of current from a high frequency unit is small although the voltage is very high. The overall power is quite low.*

POINTS TO NOTE ▷

- With *high frequency the current disperses into the client's body at the point of contact.*
- *As the effects are concentrated around the electrode they are superficial, but care must be taken when sparking not to over-treat as this can lead to over desquamation and drying of the skin during subsequent days.*

PROGRESS CHECK

1 Give four examples of vacuum applicators and in each case briefly outline their purpose.
2 List ten contraindications to vacuum suction.
3 State four reasons for giving a vacuum suction treatment.
4 Describe a high frequency current.
5 Name and describe the two different treatments that can be given using the high frequency machine.

Neuro-muscular electrical stimulation (NMES)

This treatment is referred to by many different names such as electrical muscle stimulation (EMS), faradic (after the original type of current used for muscle stimulation), or by manufacturers' trade names, e.g. Slendertone^{TM}. It is used to improve and maintain muscular tone and is a passive form of exercise as the client lies and relaxes whilst the machine emits electrical impulses to stimulate the muscles' motor nerves to bring about muscle contraction. To be effective the treatment has to be part of a course to develop the full effect within the muscles. It is extremely beneficial for clients who do not enjoy physical exercise or who are contraindicated to strenuous exercise or for those wishing to tone particular muscle groups, e.g. abdominals for post natal mothers.

Fig. 6.26 *Neuro-muscular electrical stimulation*

192

POINT TO NOTE ▷ *A course of NMES treatment will improve the client's shape and inch loss will usually be noted.*

NMES machines use an interrupted direct current of a low frequency which is released into the body via a conductive electrode which is connected to the faradic unit via electrical leads. The majority of machines offer the therapist the facility to use the equipment on both face and body by using different electrodes and by varying the parameters of the current. Machines, however, are available for just face or body. Faradic treatments have been extremely popular for figure improvement programmes particularly when combined with other salon treatments such as gyratory massage and galvanic along with home care advice on diet and exercise. In recent years there has been great technological advancement by equipment manufacturers who have developed and adapted faradic currents to develop more specialised salon treatments for figure improvement (see Chapter 7).

NMES units generally have the following controls:

- A mains switch for turning the unit on or off. This is often combined with a timer.
- A safety aspect on most modern machines is a reset feature which prevents the machine working if any of the electrode outlet dials are not at zero.
- Intensity dials for each electrode outlet. As these dials are increased, so is the intensity of the current flowing through the electrodes.
- Contraction (surge or stimulation period) and relaxation dials which enable the therapist to select the appropriate times to suit the area of the body being treated and the existing condition of the client's muscle.
- A pulse sequence, wave form or phasic control. On the majority of equipment only two types are found; mono-phasic and bi-phasic. Mono-phasic emits pulses flowing in one direction only. Bi-phasic emits pulses flowing in both directions; back and forth or negative to positive then positive to negative. The other selections available either on this dial or as a separate mode dial are:

  Mono-phasic on a regular basis. Pulses are emitted as per the machine setting, e.g. contracting for 2 seconds and relaxing for 2.5 seconds.

  Bi-phasic on a regular basis. Pulses are emitted as per the machine setting.

  Mono-phasic and bi-phasic on an irregular basis. With this setting the machine is programmed to alter the pattern of the set contraction and relaxation time. This is particularly useful when a client is a little apprehensive of the treatment and tends to automatically tighten their muscles when they expect the contraction to occur. It is also useful to add variety to the treatment for a regular client.

- A frequency dial. This enables the therapist to select the number of pulses per second emitted from the machine to stimulate the motor points. Traditionally for superficial muscles, such as those of the face,

193

120 is used whereas for deeper work on large muscles between 60–90 is used. However the most recent research has shown a wider application of frequency is beneficial, especially when recreating passive exercise most closely similar to physical activity.

* A pulse width. This changes the actual width of each pulse emitted (the length of time it stays in the muscle). The higher the setting of this dial the greater the effect to the muscle. For facial muscles a lower setting is usually used, e.g. 80 μs, whereas on the large body muscles a higher setting is required, e.g. from 160 μs upwards and if the client has a lot of adipose tissue the dial may be started at a higher setting still, such as 240 μs.

* Some machines have a master output control which can increase the percentage intensity of current to all the electrodes in use without turning them up individually.

* Pulse envelope control. Usually only available on more specialised units, this controls the configuration of pulses in the contraction time. It is adjusted to enable more comfortable, effective contractions.

GOOD PRACTICE ▷ *Care must be taken not to over work the muscles.*

Electrodes

There is a wide variety of electrodes available for use with faradic-type machines. To enable the current to flow to stimulate the muscles a positive electrode (anode) and negative electrode (cathode) are needed.

The most widely used modern faradic electrodes for application of the current to the body are rubber pads which are impregnated with an electrical conductor such as carbon on one side. These pads can vary in shape and size but are used in pairs to enable the current to flow from one to the other.

For facial treatments there are three types of electrode available for use:

* Facial block electrode (dual head). The most popular type manufactured and used which houses the anode and cathode in its insulated holder. They vary in form and in use, e.g. some have an in-built intensity control to adapt the current easily, the distance between the anode and cathode may be fixed or if the electrode has a stylus the therapist can alter the distance between these. They are ideal for stimulating a number of motor points which are situated closely together on the face.

* Mushroom electrode (disc electrode). A metal disc in the electrode must be covered in several layers of lint to protect the client. The *indifferent electrode* is protected with a foam pouch and is placed in contact with the client's body by either lying it under the shoulder or, as with some machines, by using a wrist clip. The mushroom head is placed on the motor point of the muscle, acting as the *active electrode* and completing the electrical circuit.

USEFUL INFORMATION

The mushroom electrode is not particularly used in salons but has traditionally been used by colleges.

* Mask electrode. This houses a variety of electrodes inside to stimulate all the muscles of the face at the same time. This would not be used on claustrophobic clients.

Types of padding

The selection of the padding method for treatment will be dependent on a number of things:

* The phase control to be used. With bi-phasic the current is even from the positive and negative electrodes whereas with mono-phasic the current is stronger from the negative electrode.
* The areas to be treated and the number of pairs of electrodes available, e.g. if there are a large number of muscles to stimulate there may be insufficient electrodes to use the longitudinal method and therefore split padding may have to be used.
* Manufacturers instructions. These should always be followed carefully as the manufacturers will recommend the most suitable type of padding to gain maximum benefit from their machine.

Longitudinal padding

Modern longitudinal padding involves placing the anode and cathode on to the top and bottom motor points of the same muscle, e.g. rectus abdominus, triceps, rectus femoris, etc., bringing about a smoother, even contraction. This term was used to describe the padding of the origin and insertion of a muscle whereby the current had to flow via the motor point to bring about a contraction. Modern longitudinal padding usually refers to the placing of the electrodes on to a muscle with two motor points.

Dual or duplicate padding

This type of padding involves using the anode and cathode of a pair of pads on one or two muscles on one side of the body and then placing another pair on the adjacent muscle group, e.g. the obliques, rectus abdominus, adductors, abductors, etc.

Split padding

With this type of padding a pair of pads is split and placed on the same muscle group on opposite sides of the body, e.g. gluteus maximus, pectorals, etc.

POINT TO NOTE ▷
- *With split padding you cannot alter the intensity if one side is weaker than the other.*
- *With split padding the bi-phasic mode must be selected.*

ACTIVITY

With a colleague carry out three different body NMES treatments using the different methods of padding. Discuss the effectiveness and comfort of each method.

CONTRAINDICATIONS

to NMES

! Disorders of the nervous system.

! Disorders of or injury of the muscular system.

! Loss of skin sensation.

! Recent scar tissue.

! Broken bones.

! Hypersensitive skins.

! Heart conditions.

! Pacemakers.

! High or low blood pressure.*

! Thrombosis or phlebitis.

! Highly apprehensive clients.

! Epilepsy.*

! Diabetes.*

! Migraine sufferers.

! Cuts and abrasions.

! Highly vascular conditions.

! Metal plates, pins, bridges, IUD or if the client has an excessive amount of fillings.

! Over bony areas.

! Pregnancy.**

* Only to be carried out with medical approval.

**Exclude the abdomen.

Effects of NMES

- Stimulates the nerves and causes muscle contraction which acts as a passive form of exercise to strengthen and tone muscles.
- Increases blood circulation.

Reasons for using NMES

* To strengthen and tone poor muscles, e.g. abdominal and pectorals of post natal mothers.
* To improve the contours of the face and body, e.g. platysma, abdominal, gluteals.
* To assist in tightening muscles after weight loss.
* To assist in improving a client's posture by stretching and toning shortened muscles, e.g. pectorals in kyphosis.

Preparation for NMES treatment

1 Observe general safety precautions for using electrical equipment.

2 The machine is placed on a stable trolley.

3 The machine is checked and tested by the therapist to ensure it is working correctly.

4 The products required for treatment are selected and placed on the trolley.

NMES Treatment

1 Client is greeted at reception and escorted to treatment area.

2 Consultation is carried out to check for contraindications and to explain the effects of the treatment. A skin sensitivity test is carried out on the area to be treated.

Note. If performing a body treatment, the client's measurements can be noted prior to treatment.

3 Client removes their jewellery, showers and may have a heat treatment to relax the muscles prior to treatment and/or an additional salon treatment, e.g. gyratory massage.

4 Client is helped onto the couch.

5 The therapist ensures the client is warm and comfortable.

6 The skin is free of grease as this would act as a barrier to the current and prevent a good contraction.

7 The therapist tests the machine in front of the client.

8 If treating the body, elasticated straps are wrapped and firmly secured around the area to be treated.

9 Having considered the client's needs and the machine being used, the therapist selects an appropriate method of padding, dampens the electrodes with warm water or conductive gel and places them firmly in contact with the client's skin.

Method

1 Ensure mains lead is plugged in to mains supply and that all switches are off and all dials are at zero.

Pectoralis
Pectoralis positive pad(+) place under arm

External oblique

Rectus abdominis

Vastus lateralis

Gracilis

Rectus femoris

Anterior

Trapezius

Biceps

Latissimus dorsi

Gluteus maximus

Biceps femoris

Gastrocnemius

Posterior

Fig. 6.27 *Example of faradic padding on the biphasic mode*

2 The therapist selects the appropriate treatment time, contraction and relaxation period, the mode, pulse sequence and width.

3 If performing a facial treatment the therapist dampens the facial electrode and places it firmly in contact with the treatment area.

Note. If using the mushroom electrode, the therapist first places the indifferent electrode firmly in contact with the client's skin (behind the shoulder or strapped to the wrist). If using a mask electrode it is firmly strapped around the client's face and neck and as the electrodes are simultaneously activated by the intensity dial the therapist would check on client sensation and comfort until contractions were achieved. The treatment time would begin at around 8 minutes and build throughout the course of treatments to 15 minutes.

4 The therapist slowly turns up the intensity dial during the contraction time only, checking with the client on how it feels.

GOOD PRACTICE ▷

* *It is very important to use a good conductive medium.*
* *If working on the body all electrodes need to be turned up individually until the client feels a slight tingling sensation. By doing this it allows the client time to relax and adjust to the treatment before the therapist turns the individual intensity dials to achieve a contraction.*

POINT TO NOTE ▷ *Some machines allow the therapist to increase the intensity during the treatment to all electrodes by adjusting the master output dial.*

When working on the face, neck and décolleté areas it is advisable to contract the muscle 6–8 times before switching the intensity dial off during the relaxation period and moving the electrode to the next muscle. The sequence is then repeated two or three times throughout the course of treatments.

When working on the body the therapist must ensure even contractions are achieved on all the muscles being worked. If a muscle is weaker it will need a lower intensity to a stronger more toned muscle. The treatment time is usually around 20–40 minutes depending upon the treatment effects and condition. It is important to ensure that the client is warm and comfortable throughout the treatment.

5 At the end of the treatment the therapist ensures all dials are switched off before removing the electrodes. It is advisable to turn the intensity control down during the relaxation period.

6 If recommended, further treatment may be given.

7 The client is helped from the couch, the record card completed (if performing a body treatment the client's measurements may be recorded), appropriate home care and further salon treatment advice is given (with faradic treatment it is recommended that a client has a minimum of two to three sessions per week for six to eight weeks) along with samples of any skin care products used and the client's next appointment is confirmed.

8 The therapist tidies the treatment area and cleans the electrodes used by carefully wiping with hot water and detergent.

USEFUL INFORMATION

Saline solution used to be applied to the electrodes as a conductor but most manufacturers today feel that there are sufficient mineral salts present in tap water to act as a conductor.

USEFUL INFORMATION

Faradic pads deteriorate with use and become less conductive so will need replacing regularly.

POINTS TO NOTE ▷ *Poor contraction of muscles may be due to:*

- *Any grease left on the skin.*
- *The electrodes are too dry (they may need re-damping during the treatment).*
- *The electrodes are not firmly in contact with the skin.*
- *The intensity selected is too low.*
- *The pulse frequency and width are not set correctly.*
- *Trying to stimulate muscles through large quantities of adipose tissue which can act as a barrier to the current.*
- *Incorrect positioning of the electrodes. It is important to switch the intensity dial to zero before moving the pads.*
- *Faulty connections on the machine or leads. The leads need regular checking and maintenance.*
- *Muscle fatigue.*

Galvanic

Galvanic treatments have become extremely popular over the last few years. The current brings about chemical and physical reactions within the body and it is commercially used with professional products to improve the client's face and body appearance. There are a wide variety of gels and ampoules manufactured and recommended for different skin types and conditions.

The galvanic machine can be applied with the appropriate products to offer two treatments to the client:

- Desincrustation – this is given to deep cleanse the skin.
- Iontophoresis – this is used to introduce beneficial ingredients into the skin for particular skin types or conditions, e.g. oily, dry or couperose skins.

Galvanic treatment is used on the body to assist in the dispersal of cellulite.

POINT TO NOTE ▷ *The range of products available include gel and ampoule preparations and specially formulated solutions.*

The principles of the galvanic treatment for face and body is the same but the application, products used, treatment time, further salon treatment and home care advice are different. The machines use a direct current of a low voltage. They can be purchased for face or body work individually or combined in a face and body unit or in a combined unit with another electrical treatment such as high frequency. This last combination is commonly found in salons as these two treatments are popularly used with professional products for improved skin care (see Chapter 7).

Galvanic units consist of:

- A mains control switch which may be connected to a timer
- Outlets for connecting the electrodes which are used in pairs (anode and cathode)
- Intensity dial and milliamp meter for registering the amount of current applied (and indirectly to indicate the level of the client's skin resistance).
- Polarity switch.

It is *extremely important that the therapist reads and follows the manufacturers instructions* as although there is a standard understanding that the red wire of an electrode is positive and the black lead is negative, most manufacturers have adapted their machines to enable the therapist to reverse the polarity of the leads at a flick of a switch which could easily cause confusion if the manufacturers instructions are not read.

The therapist must fully understand their unit and if terms such as 'normal' and 'reverse' are indicated, know accurately how this refers to the polarity of the leads and outlets. Usually this is a simple point to clarify, but it should not be assumed as manufacturers vary in the use of

USEFUL INFORMATION

The type of product, its viscosity, etc., will determine the most appropriate method of application. Each product will list the most active ingredients for a specific purpose, i.e. products for couperose skins tend to contain a vasoconstrictor such as horse chestnut.

terminology and presentation, i.e. some units have separate outlets for the anode and cathode and others are coupled.

The intensity of the output is measured in milliamps and can be registered on either:

* a moving coil meter, i.e. a gauge with an arm
* a LED (light emitting diode)
* a LCD (liquid crystal display).

For facial therapy treatment, intensity settings are low and indicated by the product directive and the type of skin being treated. Ranges between 0.2–0.6 mA are common, but individual sensory responses are an important factor to be considered along with manufacturer's instructions.

For body therapy the following calculation can be used to work out the maximum milliamps current setting for a pad size:

Manufacturer's recommended maximum = 0.05 mA per square centimetre
Pad size = 11 cm × 11 cm = 121 cm^2
Maximum current setting = 121 × 0.05 = 6.05 mA

Terminology referred to in galvanic treatments

* Anode = positive electrode.
* Cathode = negative electrode.
* Active electrode = the electrode in contact with the client's face during facial treatment.
* Indifferent electrode = the electrode held by the client to complete the electrical circuit.
* Anions = negatively charged ions, used in professional products which determine the polarity of the active electrode.
* Cations = positively charged ions.
* Anaphoresis = the flow of anions to the anode.
* Cataphoresis = the flow of cations to the cathode.

The galvanic treatment operates on the basic principle that like poles repel and opposite poles attract (see Fig. 6.28). The products selected are repelled into the skin by the active electrode which must be of the same polarity as the product.

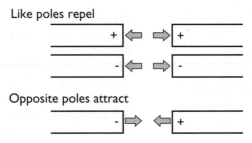

Fig. 6.28 *Like poles repel, opposites attract*

POINT TO NOTE ▷ *The polarity of the active electrode is determined by the product used so care should be taken to read the manufacturers instructions. The majority of products tend to be 'negative to positive' but the actual time for which the negative or positive poles are used will once again vary depending on the type of treatment being given and the manufacturers instructions.*

Fig. 6.29 *Anaphoresis*

Electrodes

There are a variety of electrodes available for use on the face.

Types of active electrode:

⊛ Metal rollers.

⊛ Metal ball – single/double prong.

⊛ Tweezer or flat head electrode.

Tweezers or flat head electrodes are usually covered with either dampened gauze, lint or cotton wool, according to the manufacturers instructions or worked over a gauze masque soaked in active solution.

Types of indifferent electrodes:

⊛ Metal bar. Some companies recommend that the electrode is covered in a dampened sponge pouch.

⊛ Flat plate. These are generally supplied with a sponge pouch which is dampened before application.

Body electrodes

⊛ Galvanic pads. These come in pairs, having a positive and negative electrode, and should be supplied with sponge pouches which are designed to protect against galvanic burns. The sponges are dampened prior to use and the active side of the galvanic pad is placed face down. Several layers of a lint wadding can be used instead but care must be taken to ensure an even contact is made.

Note. It is important to check that the sponge or lint layers do not dry out during treatment.

USEFUL INFORMATION

Some conductive electrodes are conductive on both sides. This is not recommended for safe body application. If these are to be used care must be taken to insulate the top of the pad before securing with elasticated straps.

POINT TO NOTE ▷ *During a facial treatment the active cathode removes the body's sebum and in doing so lowers the skin's resistance to the current, therefore it may be necessary to reduce the intensity of the current during treatment.*

GOOD PRACTICE ▷ • *Sponge pouches must be thoroughly washed after use with warm water and detergent then soaked in a suitable disinfectant and thoroughly rinsed.*

• *Sponges will deteriorate with wear and tear and must be replaced as needed.*

CONTRAINDICATIONS

to galvanic treatment

! Loss of skin sensation.

! Recent scar tissue.

! Infectious skin diseases or disorders.

! Broken bones.

! Hypersensitive skins.

! Heart conditions.

! Pacemakers.

! Low blood pressure.

! Epilepsy.*

! Diabetes.*

! Migraine sufferers.

! Cuts and abrasions.

! Highly vascular conditions.

! Metal plates, pins, bridges or an excessive amount of fillings.

! Pregnancy.*

* Only to be carried out with medical approval.

Effects of galvanic treatment

Effects at the cathode

The cathode produces an alkali effect on the skin by bringing about a chemical reaction between sodium ions and the hydroxyl ions of water to produce sodium hydroxide which is an alkali, thus creating the following effects:

• Breaks down the acid mantle.

• Relaxes the pores.

* Increases the blood circulation – vasodilation occurs.
* Hyperaemia.
* Warmth in the tissues.
* Brings about saponification – the emulsifying and removal of sebum.
* Creates a softening and drying effect on the skin.
* Stimulates nerve endings.
* Moisture is temporarily drawn to the cathode.

Effects at the anode

The anode produces an acidic effect on the skin by bringing about a chemical reaction between the chloride ions and hydrogen ions present in tap water to produce hydrochloric acid and oxygen, thus creating the following effects:

* Restores the acid mantle.
* Tightens the pores.
* Hardening of the skin.
* Creates warmth in the tissues.
* Reduces circulation.
* Soothing effect on the nerve endings, if used for a short time.

ACTIVITY

Research the variety of products available for use with galvanic equipment. Consider their size, cost, ingredients and usage.

POINTS TO NOTE ▷

* *Care should be taken when using galvanic treatments, particularly with treatment to the body as if too high an intensity of current is used or the duration of the treatment is too long or skin sensitivity has not been accurately diagnosed or insufficient insulation is used, it may cause a galvanic burn which can be a mixture of a chemical and over-heating reaction.*
* *Galvanic burns are extremely painful and take a very long time to heal. They generally appear under the cathode and will initially look red and will later turn grey and weep.*

GOOD PRACTICE ▷

* *The therapist should always remain with a client during galvanic treatments and check on their comfort continually.*
* *It is essential for all galvanic treatments that a good and even conduction is achieved at all times.*

Reasons for using galvanic treatment

* To deep cleanse the skin.
* To introduce active ingredients to benefit the client's skin condition.
* To assist in dispersing cellulite.

Preparation for galvanic treatment

1 Observe general safety precautions for using electrical equipment.

2 The machine is placed on a stable trolley.

3 The machine is checked and tested by the therapist to ensure it is working correctly.

4 The products required for treatment are selected and placed on the trolley.

Galvanic treatment to the face and neck

1 Client is greeted at reception and escorted to treatment area.

2 Consultation is carried out to check for contraindications and to explain the effects of the treatment. A skin sensitivity test is carried out on the area to be treated.

3 Client removes their jewellery.

4 Client is helped onto the couch and their clothing and hair protected.

5 The therapist ensures the client is warm and comfortable.

6 The skin is cleansed with suitable products and if using a cream based product the therapist must ensure that there is no residue left on the skin which would act as a barrier to the current.

Note. A vapouriser can be used to soften the skin and lower the client's skin resistance. There are also a variety of conductive lotions available that may be used.

7 A suitable medium is selected and applied to the client's face and neck, e.g. desincrustation gel or active ampoule. It is usually recommended that ampoules are applied with a gauze masque rather than directly on to the skin.

Note. The type of product selected for facial work will influence the type of electrode used, e.g. metal roller and ball electrodes tend to be used with gels whereas the other electrodes tend to be used with ampoules.

Method

1 Ensure mains lead is plugged in to mains supply and that all switches are off and all dials are at zero.

2 The therapist tests the machine in front of the client and explains its use.

3 The selected electrodes are wiped with disinfectant and prepared for use according to manufacturers instructions.

4 The therapist ensures the electrodes are correctly fitted and that the correct polarity for the product being used is selected.

5 Depending on the type of indifferent electrode being used, it is either given to the client to hold firmly or is placed under the client's shoulder or clipped to the client's arm.

USEFUL INFORMATION

Japanese galvanic equipment tends to include the arm clip indifferent electrode.

6 The therapist places the selected active electrode in contact with the client's skin and moves it around using small movements whilst turning the mains control switch on and the intensity dial up according to the manufacturers instructions. Do not begin treatment on the forehead or around the eyes.

Note. The client is advised that they may get a metallic taste in the mouth if they have fillings whilst working around the mouth and nose area. Some clients feel a slight warmth in the tissues, others don't feel any reaction, but do not be tempted to increase the milliamp intensity beyond recommended levels as blood vessels can dilate and if there is insufficient product on the skin a galvanic (chemical) burn could result. Ensure that the machine is working correctly and any manufacturers instructions for equipment/product are being followed.

7 The therapist moves the active electrode slowly over the client's face and neck in a methodical pattern. The treatment time will vary according to the type of treatment being given, the skin condition and the manufacturers instructions, so it is essential that the therapist studies these carefully. Carlton Professional recommend the following for use with their products and equipment:

> Desincrustation – 15–20 minutes negative to positive.
>
> Iontophoresis – 5–7 minutes negative to positive.

The positive polarity is generally used for the final 2–3 minutes.

It is important that the therapist keeps the active electrode moving and in contact with the skin whilst turning the intensity dial to zero before removing the electrode from the skin to reverse the polarity.

8 At the end of the treatment the therapist ensures all dials are set to zero and switched off before removing the electrodes.

9 The selected medium is removed and further treatment, such as facial massage or direct high frequency, may be given or the skin is toned and moisturised.

10 The client is helped from the couch, the record card completed, appropriate home care and further salon treatment advice is given, along with samples of the skin care products used and the client's next appointment is confirmed.

11 The therapist tidies the treatment area and cleans the electrodes used by carefully wiping with hot water and disinfectant.

Galvanic treatment to the body

1 Client is greeted at reception and escorted to treatment area.

2 Consultation is carried out to check for contraindications and to explain the effects of the treatment. A skin sensitivity test is carried out on the area to be treated.

3 Client removes their jewellery, showers and may have a mild heat treatment to relax the tissues prior to treatment and/or an additional salon treatment such as gyratory massage.

Fig. 6.30 *Super Galvanic equipment*

4 Client is helped onto the couch.

5 The therapist ensures the client is warm and comfortable.

6 The therapist ensures the skin is free of grease as this would act as a barrier to the current.

7 The therapist tests the machine in front of the client and checks all leads are providing a working circuit.

POINT TO NOTE ⊳ *Prior to treatment mild sudation is recommended, but not any excessive sweating.*

Method
1 Ensure mains lead is plugged in to mains supply and that all switches are off and all dials are at zero.

2 Elasticated body straps are wrapped firmly around the area to be treated. The therapist applies the selected product, e.g. cellulite gel or ampoule to the skin/sponge pouch and places the insulated electrodes according to manufactures instructions. (If the electrodes are conductive on both sides ensure the top surface is insulated before fixing with elasticated strapping). In treatment for cellulite the stronger, active, cathode pads are placed on the main cellulite areas whilst the anode is generally placed parallel or opposite.

3 The therapist ensures the electrodes are correctly fitted and that the correct polarity for the product being used is selected.

4 The intensity dials are turned up individually until either the client feels a slight tingling sensation, or until the maximum output recommended is reached.

Posterior   Anterior

Fig. 6.31   *Example of galvanic padding*

5 The treatment time may take up to approximately 20 minutes according to the client's tolerance. The polarity is generally reversed for the last 3–5 minutes of the treatment.

6 At the end of the treatment, or in between changing polarity, the therapist must turn the intensity dial to zero before switching off the machine and removing the insulated electrodes from the skin.

7 The selected medium is removed and further treatment such as NMES may be given. Care should be taken in any subsequent pad and product placement to avoid over irritation or stimulation.

8 The client is helped from the couch, the record card completed, appropriate home care and further salon treatment advice is given and the client's next appointment is confirmed.

Note. For treatment of cellulite it is recommended that the client has a minimum of 2–3 sessions per week with a total number of 12 treatments before a significant difference can be seen.

9 The therapist tidies the treatment area and cleans the electrodes used by carefully wiping with hot water and then disinfectant.

POINTS TO NOTE ▷
* For treatment of cellulite, diet and exercise should be combined with body galvanic treatments.
* The client's cellulite condition can often appear worse before improvement is seen due to the redistribution of fatty fluids in the area.
* Body galvanic treatment helps to relax and loosen the adipose tissues and waste elements that bring about cellulite. It is not effective as a treatment on its own.

ACTIVITY

1 Identify three clients with differing skin conditions, design individual treatment programmes for them using electrical equipment. Carry out the treatments keeping a record of the products and equipment used, duration of each treatment, home care, the clients' views and evaluate the effectiveness of the programmes.

2 With a colleague design and carry out a programme, including the use of electrical equipment, to assist with figure improvement. Keep a record of the treatments and home care and evaluate the effectiveness of the programme.

Vapouriser

For years vapourisers have been used to prepare a client's skin for further treatment, such as prior to a cleansing face mask or galvanic treatments. The warmth of the vapour relaxes the tissues and softens the skin. It may also induce slight perspiration which has a cleansing action on the skin and the warmth will stimulate the sudoriferous glands thus assisting in the elimination of waste. There are a variety of vapourisers available including mobile free standing units with height adjustment facility and portable machines that are easily transported and sit on a sturdy trolley or table top. Usually distilled water is placed inside the unit and is heated by the internal heating element until a fine spray of vapour flows through the vapour jet. Most manufactures have designed units with a safety device; either a device to warn the therapist that the water level is low, or a cut-out switch to prevent the unit boiling dry. Most vapourisers have an optional ozone switch enabling the therapist to combine vapour

USEFUL INFORMATION

Ozone is produced when the vapour passes over the high pressure mercury lamp which turns the available oxygen to ozone.

Fig. 6.32 *Vapouriser*

with ozone which has a anti-bacterial effect on the skin and is therefore particularly beneficial for congested skins or after extraction work has been carried out. Vapourisers are used for differing lengths of time and from different distances from the skin according to the desired effect and overall treatment programme.

POINTS TO NOTE ▷

- *Health and Safety legislation recommends that the maximum safety level for ozone released from vapouriser units should not exceed 0.1 p.p.m. (part per million) calculated as an eight hour time-weighted average. If for example the quantity of ozone produced at a distance of 30 cm from the steamer head over an eight hour period is 0.1 p.p.m., which, if divided by eight, gives a reading for continual use of the vapouriser for one hour of 0.0125 p.p.m. This would indicate that the steamer is operating well within the recommended safety level.*

- *A traditional vapouriser has a deliberate warmth to the vapour as well as a stimulating action. Another system known as a pulveriser (favoured in France) could be confused with a vapouriser, but in this instance the vapour jet is very fast and furious and designed to apply cool, wet product to the skin.*

GOOD PRACTICE ▷

- *To maintain vapourisers in good working order they will occasionally need to be de-scaled according to the manufacturer's instructions.*

- *Do not use if the vapouriser is spitting hot water: check that the kettle is not overfilled or that there is not a blockage in the jet outlet (refer to the maintenance manual).*

- *Some vapourisers are designed to enable the therapist to infuse essential oils to suit the individual client.*

CONTRAINDICATIONS

to using a vapouriser

! Highly vascular conditions.

! Sunburn.

! Acne rosacea.

Brush cleansing

Brush cleansing machines are used to aid the desquamation of the skin and to aid cellular regeneration by stimulating the skin's blood circulation. They can be used to give a deep cleansing of the skin, to aid in the removal of peels or masks or to give a stimulating massage. The units are supplied with a variety of massage heads allowing the therapist to select the appropriate head according to the client's skin type and the desired effects of the treatment. The machine have a mains on/off switch and a variable speed control and some incorporate a directional control

Fig. 6.33 *Brush cleansing equipment*

to enable the therapist at a turn of a dial to ensure the skin is being lifted rather than pulled down. If the machine is being used for cleansing or massage, suitable water-based foaming products should be used to facilitate the action of the massage heads. The circular, rotating heads should be applied to the skin dampened and flat to the skin, i.e. making a right angle between skin and handle.

CONTRAINDICATIONS

to brush cleansing

! Skin diseases or disorders.

! Hyper sensitive skin.

! Extremely loose skin tissue.

! Cuts or abrasions.

! Diabetes.*

! Highly vascular conditions.

! Any skin inflammation.

! Recent scar tissue.

! Sunburn.

* Only to be carried out with medical approval.

POINTS TO NOTE ▷
* Brushing can be used for lymph stimulation massage. The direction of the massage head should be 'lifting' the skin.
* Treatment time is on average 5–7 minutes.

PROGRESS CHECK

1 State the different types of electrical treatments for:
   a the face
   b the body.
2 Describe the general effects of the following treatments:
   a neuro-mulscular electrical stimulation
   b desincrustation
   c iontophoresis
   d vapourisers
   e brush cleanse.

3 List four contraindications for each of the following treatments:
  a neuro-muscular electrical stimulation
  b facial galvanic treatments
  c vapourisers
  d brush cleanse.

4 Describe the electrical currents used in the following treatments:
  a neuro-muscular electrical stimulation
  b galvanic

5 Explain the following terms:
  a anode
  b cathode
  c anion
  d cation.

— KEY TERMS —

You need to know what these words and phrases mean. Go back through the chapter to find out.

Care of electrical equipment
Safety precautions
Skin sensitivity test
Mechanical massagers
Vacuum suction massage
High frequency

Neuro-muscular electrical stimulation (NMES)
Galvanic
Vapourisers
Brush cleansing

7 Specialised salon treatments for figure and skin improvement

After working through this chapter you will be able to:

➤ identify the different specialised treatments available

➤ describe the benefits of the specialised treatments.

As with all specialised salon treatments, it is essential to research the companies' products and equipment, the effects, potential market and growth of the treatments. It is important to note that with these specialised salon treatments the therapist must undertake all necessary training from the manufacturer/agent concerned.

Manual treatments

Manual cellulite treatments

A number of professional skin care companies offer specialised manual treatments that aim to reduce and improve the appearance of cellulite. They normally work in two ways, either by the action of the product itself or the massage techniques used.

Products

There are certain ingredients, in particular plant extracts and essential oils, that are known to have an effect on cellulite. Examples of these include:

* Essential oil of rosemary – this has a tonic effect and is anti-toxic.
* Essential oil of sandalwood– eliminates toxins and decongests.
* Essential oil of patchouli – this has a regenerative effect and is healing.
* Essential oil of lavender – this has a healing and diuretic effect.
* Seaweed – acts as a diuretic
* Horsetail extract – tonic action on the tissues.

Massage techniques

These often incorporate specialised movements that help in lymphatic drainage and compression type movements as the circulation is reduced in these areas and needs improving if effective elimination is going to take place.

For any of the cellulite treatments to be successful they need to be given in courses with proper home care advice. The client should be encouraged to look at diet and eliminate convenience-type foods, too much salt, sugar, tea, coffee, etc., and to look at lifestyle; in particular smoking, alcohol consumption and exercise.

The client must be able to attend the clinic a least two to three times a week for a course of treatments lasting from 20 to 30 minutes on average. The client must also be prepared to invest in products to be used at home in between salon visits and to use them daily.

Example of a cellulite treatment.

1 Perform a detailed consultation, checking the area for any contra-indications.

2 Prepare the client for treatment ensuring comfort throughout.

3 Uncover the area and clean with specialised toning product.

4 Apply exfoliating cream evenly to the treatment area, remove when dry using circular movements. Support the skin as required.

5 Wipe area with toner to remove any residual cream.

6 Apply cellulite treatment oil and massage the area using lymphatic drainage movements and compression techniques.

7 Apply specialised cellulite gel/serum and work into the area.

8 Often some form of heat is next applied to the area to help the absorption of the products; it may be in the form of cellophane sheeting, a warm poultice or a thermal blanket.

9 Remove the thermal medium and any traces of residual product.

10 Apply cellulite cream and massage into area.

11 Recommend home care advice and book the next treatment.

Products for home care

Home care normally consists of using some kind of cellulite serum/gel and cream which needs to be applied daily, preferably morning and at night, and usually following a brisk circulatory massage.

Stretch Marks

These treatments aim to reactivate the dermis and increase the localised circulation. Success of the treatment will depend on regular salon treatment (2–3 times per week) over a course of 12–20 on average.The client will also need to purchase homecare products to be used in between salon visits.

Common ingredients used in stretch mark treatments include plant extracts and essential oils. For example:

- Hops – have a firming and tightening effect.
- Ginseng – aids cellular stimulation and has an anti-ageing effect.
- Horsetail – restores elasticity in fibres and collagen of the skin.
- Essential oil of mint – tones, firms and increases circulation.

Example of a stretch mark treatment.

1 Perform a thorough consultation, checking the area for any contra-indications and make sure that the stretch marks are at a stage where they will respond to treatment.

2 Wipe over the area with toner and exfoliate to remove dead skin cells to allow easier absorption of products.

3 Next stimulate the area to be treated with either a body brush, body mitten, specific equipment or even brisk effleurage type movements.

4 Apply a specialised stretch mark gel/solution and work it into the area briskly.

5 A stimulating product is applied and massaged it into the area. The massage sequence should be quite brisk and include pinching type movements, e.g. Jacquet.

6 Thermal equipment/product can be applied to allow the active solutions to penetrate more thoroughly.

8 Remove any residue of products.

9 Finally prescribe the most appropriate products for the upkeep of the skin at home and book the next treatment.

Skin improvement treatments

One of the latest advances in skin improvement has been the development of skin renewal treatments. On the surface it may seem that nothing is new, peeling products have been used for a long time – even as far back as Egyptian times. As recently as 1927 chemical peels were used to dissolve dead skin tissue. However in the last few years two substances have been generating media interest. They are retinoic acid and alpha hydroxy acid (AHA).

Retinoic Acid

Retinoic acid is Vitamin A and was originally developed as a formulation for the treatment of acne vulgaris. It was found to speed up the natural shedding of the epidermis and recent trials have shown it to be very effective (if used in low concentrations) on sun damage, ageing, fine lines and wrinkles and pigmentation. However it does need to be used for six months and once discontinued, stops working. There can be side effects however and a lot of people develop residual inflammation as the treatment reduces the thickness of the stratum corneum.

This is not performed as a salon treatment, clients usually obtain the retinoic acid on prescription. Beauty therapists need to take great care with any client using retinoic acid products. In particular avoid waxing, peeling or extracting in areas being treated.

Alpha hydroxy acids (AHA)

These are also sometimes referred to as fruit acids and were developed following the interest in retinoic acid.

They work by causing micro-exfoliation which speeds up the natural exfoliation process of the skin. Some of the ingredients literally digest the surface cells therefore revealing new skin. This is a very important concept in the treatment of the skin as many problems that occur are the result of a build up of dead skin cells or *hyperkeritinisation* as it is technically known.

Great care should be taken with the use and administration of these products however as they can be extremely harsh if not used in the correct quantity.

Some key ingredients used in AHA creams are:

- **Lactic acid.** This alpha hydroxy acid occurs naturally in sour milk and dissolves the intercellular cement holding the skin cells together. It also works on follicular skin cells helping dislodge blockages and therefore helping prevent congestion.
- **Glycolic acid.** This is used for its small molecular structure as it is able to penetrate quickly and deeply and dissolves the natural moisturising factor of the skin. It can cause more irritation than lactic acid.
- **Salicylic adic.** This stimulates the formation of new epidermal skin cells in the stratum germinativum and has antiseptic properties
- **Bromelain.** This is a pineapple derivative and is a fruit enzyme that digests surface skin cells.
- **Papain.** This comes from the papaya fruit and is an enzyme. It again digests the surface skin cells.
- **Citric acid.** This is derived from citrus fruits and is also a fruit enzyme that digests the surface skin cells.
- **Plant and flower extracts.** Examples include orange flower, aloe vera and cornflower. They are added for their soothing and hydrating properties.

Buffers

Alpha hydroxy acid treatments have a buffer added to make them less aggressive in reaction on the skin. Plant extracts and enzymes are used as buffers and they have the effect of altering the pH of reaction.

AHA treatments exist in two forms; a concentrated strength for use by the therapist in the clinic and a lower concentration for the client to use at home daily between salon visits. The combination of the professional and the home care products will achieve the most rapid improvement in the appearance of the skin and as a general guide most manufacturers recommend a course of at least six salon treatments to be taken once a week initially with the daily use of homecare products.

Example of an AHA facial treatment

1 Perform a detailed consultation checking the area for any contra-indications.

2 Remove the eye and lip make-up with a suitable product making sure there is no residue left on the skin.

3 Next cleanse the face and neck with an appropriate cleanser at least twice and again thoroughly remove.

4 The special fruit acid solution is applied to the skin and left on according to individual manufacturer's instructions.

5 After the correct time the product is removed very thoroughly, usually with sponges and copious amounts of warm water, making sure no residue is left.

6 Extractions can now be performed where necessary.

7 The skin is massaged with a special soothing product to help calm the skin and reduce irritation.

8 A soothing mask is applied.

9 A special toner is applied often by means of a 'spray' action.

10 Finally a protective cream is applied to filter ultra-violet rays and nourish the skin.

11 To conclude the treatment the therapist explains the relevant homecare and retail advice and confirms the date of the next appointment.

POINT TO NOTE ▷ *Some clients may feel mild tingling or itching whilst having AHA treatments and the skin may even be pink for a short time afterwards. This is a normal reaction and must be clearly explained to the client. However, in extreme cases an abnormal reaction may occur in which case treatment should be discontinued.*

GOOD PRACTICE ▷ *Many manufacturers recommend some form of patch testing of products before commencing treatments and also a preparation product for the client to use at home prior to embarking on the course.*

Body wraps

Body wraps have been used in the professional beauty market for a number of years in varying forms. Most are marketed as a 'slimming treatment' as body tissues are compressed and slight fluid loss will result in inch loss together with a slight weight decrease. Body wraps offer other benefits such as cleansing the skin, tightening loose tissue, detoxifying the body, revitalising and helping improve cellulite and stretch marks.

Body wraps normally consist of three principles;

* Specialised products that contain active ingredients designed to be absorbed by the skin and aid in the elimination process. Examples of key ingredients most commonly used are seaweed – used for its diuretic effect, mineral extracts – used to nourish the skin and oceanic clay which acts as a poultice to draw toxins from the body.

* A wrapping medium – these can be almost like elastic bandages or even be some form of plastic or rubber sheeting.

217

Fig. 7.1 *Body wrap treatment*

⊛ Thermal activity. This can be in the form of a heat treatment – infra-red lamps or a thermal blanket – and is designed to keep the client warm as the wrapping medium and products cool. Some manufacturers suggest exercises to keep warm and to help with toning the body at the same time.

Most body wrap treatments are designed to be taken in courses attended regularly together with home care products and diet and exercise advice.

Example of a body wrap treatment.

1 A detailed consultation is carried out with the client checking for any contraindications and the client is weighed and measured.

2 Specific measurements are marked to show the client exactly where the tape measure was placed.

3 The wrapping medium is prepared, in particular bandages are normally soaked in a special 'clay' solution. (This should be done before the client arrives).

4 The client is then wrapped in the bandages/wrapping medium and most manufacturers suggest that the bandages are applied upwards in line with venous return. Particular attention should be observed to wrapping the back so as to offer lumbar support.

5 Extra amounts of the product are sometimes added for specific areas.

6 Once all the bandages/wrapping medium are in place, check with the client that they feel comfortable.

7 A thermal device is used to keep the client warm while the bandages cool. During treatment time it also induces relaxation. Some manufacturers recommend gentle exercise or the use of a toning table. (In this case the client will normally wear some form of protective tracksuit)

8 After approximately one hour the bandages/wrapping medium are removed and the client is remeasured. Some manufacturers recommend taking a shower to remove traces of product left on the skin, some products will have been completely absorbed and a shower is not necessary.

9 Finally, recommend homecare and retail products necessary for the maintenance of the treatment and confirm the next treatment.

POINT TO NOTE ▷ *It is extremely important to receive proper training in the application of body wrapping as the technique for applying the bandages requires particular skill and should only be carried out after completing a manufacturer's recommended course.*

PROGRESS CHECK

1 Give an example of a manual cellulite treatment.
2 What is the main purpose of a stretch mark treatment?
3 Give three factors that should be considered when performing an AHA treatment.
4 What are the main benefits of a body wrap treatment and how often should it be performed?

Toning tables

Toning tables may appear to be a relatively new concept in figure correction, however early models have existed since the 1930s when they were produced for physiotherapy and rehabilitation purposes. Modern tables have quickly established themselves in the professional beauty market. They normally consist of a motorised bed-type unit with various movable sections. It is possible to purchase them in two forms; either as individual units or as a multi-function unit.

Individual units are tables designed to work on one specific area of the body and would normally be part of a group of approximately six or seven units which the client uses in a treatment session lasting approximately one hour. The obvious advantage of having individual units is that more than one client can be using the tables simultaneously. The main drawback is that a lot of space is needed because each unit measures approximately 6.5 ft by 3.5 ft. This normally means that if the salon is going to purchase individual units either it is very large, or is going to specialise in toning tables and figure correction treatments generally. This type of toning table is very popular with the health spas.

Multi-function units are beds with all the features of the individual units incorporated into them so the client does not have to move once treatment commences. This type of unit is ideal if space is a problem, but it does restrict the number of clients that can use it in any one day.

The main benefits of toning tables

Toning tables are designed to improve muscle tone, mobility and reduce inches without the use of any kind of weight. They work on the principles of both isotonic and isometric exercise.

Different tables or parts of the multi-function table produce varying movements, rhythm and speed which produces progressive resistance. This in turn strengthens muscle fibres as each fibre is shortened in length improving elasticity. Toning tables also increase body temperature by increasing blood circulation; this also helps in the removal of waste products and toxins.

Types of toning table

* **Circulation table (warm-up and cool-down).** This produces a gentle vibration which is designed to increase the circulation and relax tense muscles. It should be used at the start and the end of a treatment session. There is normally an arm bar present on this table to help in toning of the upper arms, back and chest.
* **Leg table.** This concentrates on the inner and outer thighs and gluteals, but has a toning effect on the entire leg area.
* **Sit-up table.** This works the abdominal area and it is suggested that 10 minutes on this table is the equivalent to around 80 sit-ups.

Fig. 7.2 *Toning tables*

⊛ **Stomach/hip table.** This table stretches and lifts the gluteals and works the abdomen at the same time. It will also help to improve overall posture.

⊛ **Twister table.** This table alternately lifts and raises the lower legs.

⊛ **Stretching table.** This table affects the upper body, lifting the rib cage and bust and easing tension in the upper back.

A normal treatment session will last approximately one hour with roughly ten minutes being spent on each table/function. Most beds have a control panel which allows the therapist to adjust the speed of the table according to the health and general fitness of the client.

GOOD PRACTICE ▷ *It is very important that a thorough consultation is carried out before a client is allowed to use the toning tables and that they are monitored throughout the treatment.*

POINT TO NOTE ▷ *Any client using a toning table should be suitably attired, preferably in a track-suit or leotard and they should wear socks for hygienic purposes and to prevent their feet from sticking to the covering.*

Electrical treatments

Micro-electrotherapy

The concept of micro-currents is not new. It has been used in the United States of America for over twenty years in the rehabilitation of stroke patients. It is only in the last few years however that the beauty therapy profession has converted this principle to cosmetic application as an alternative to rejuvenation by surgery.

The treatment works by sending micro-current impulses via cotton-tipped electrodes or similar into the skin and underlying muscles to speed up cellular activity, regeneration and metabolism in a way very much like the body's own bio-electrical impulses. A low current is used in the treatment with some muscles being shortened, such as those of the cheeks and chin area, to give increased contour and tone, while other muscles are lengthened, such as those on the forehead, to reduce tension and expression lines.

The current also affects the lymphatic system increasing toxic removal, together with bringing fresh, oxygen rich blood into the area of treatment.

Most machines have two probes to be used simultaneously. This allows the current to work over a larger area and is ideal for body treatments. Micro-electrotherapy is different from standard galvanic equipment in

221

that it uses variable wave-forms. The wave-forms are variable to penetrate tissues at a certain depth which allows the machine to treat specific tissues in isolation.

Although the treatment tends to be marketed as one for the more mature client, it can be used on most skin types and ages as it is very cleansing and nourishing, and as mentioned above, it can be applied to the body to improve the contour of slackened muscles.

As with any treatment, proper advice to the client is essential, in particular regarding number of sessions needed, home care and retail advice. Almost every client will need to have a course of treatments taken over a period of time to notice a lasting improvement, but the unique feature of micro-electrotherapy is that most clients will see an immediate difference after one session.

Example of a micro-lifting treatment for the face

1 A very detailed consultation is carried out with the client, checking for any contraindications and discussing appropriate products to be used.

2 The skin is thoroughly cleansed ensuring that all traces of the medium are removed.

3 A specialised gel/solution is normally applied. This often contains essential oils and prepares the area for lifting by increasing the circulation and stimulating the lymphatic system. The probes are gently worked over the area.

4 A lymphatic programme is normally applied with the probes being used to follow the direction of lymphatic drainage.

5 A lifting programme is used with the machine being set on a low frequency to work the muscles, stretching and shortening as appropriate.

6 Further programmes may now be used depending on the individual manufacturer's machine. These may include more lifting, or working on the lymphatic system.

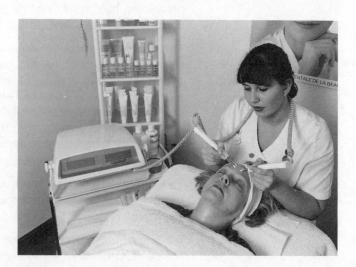

Fig. 7.3 *Facial toning treatment*

7 The treatment is normally concluded by wiping over the area to remove any residue and appying a moisturising product.

8 Relevant home care and future treatment advice should be given.

Treatment time per session for micro-electrotherapy is approximately 45 minutes to one hour.

Note. As with any toning programme it is essential that a course of treatment is given and regular maintenance thereafter.

PROGRESS CHECK

1 List the six classifications of toning table and explain the main purpose of each.
2 State the main effects of micro-electrotherapy treatments.
3 List the contraindications to specialised salon treatments.
4 What safety precautions should be observed when carrying out specialised treatments?

Specialised galvanic, high frequency and NMES treatments

Over the last decade the choice of specialised treatments has made the beauty profession one of the most innovative in existence. Modern therapy treatments have been adapted from straight forward galvanic, faradic and high frequency principles to incorporate advances in technology. Some of these treatments are designed specifically for use on the face but many are for body application. Not all are 'new' however as some are adaptions of old ideas.

Slimming treatments incorporating iontophoresis, faradic and thermal clay

This treatment is a mixture of faradic muscle stimulation and galvanic current applied in the iontophoresis mode to allow ingredients designed to help with the removal of cellulite penetrate more deeply. The treatment stimulates the circulation, aids lymphatic drainage and increases cellular activity all at the same time as toning the muscles. A special current-conducting clay is applied as this allows the treatment area to be larger and ensures even distribution of the current.

It is recommended that treatment is taken in intensive courses with products used at home in between salon visits.

POINT TO NOTE ▷ *Wet, elasticated bandages can replace the use of the clay masque and specially made flexible, conductive, black strapping can be used instead of traditional static electrodes.*

Facial treatments incorporating galvanic and high frequency treatments

These treatments are not so new and have been used in salons now for well over twenty years. They work on the principle of combining the beneficial effects of galvanic, normally the iontophoresis mode, with direct high frequency and specialised products to produce a complete treatment that is deeply cleansing, re-hydrating and increases cellular regeneration. The treatment normally lasts about one and a quarter hours and is suitable for most skin types. Cosmetic houses produce specialised products to work with the equipment and an intensive training course is usually necessary to ensure therapists adhere to correct procedures to gain maximum effect. Some manufacturers have taken the treatment a stage further and developed specialised adaptations for the eyes, neck, bust and back areas offering excellent results.

Fig. 7.4 *Cathiodermie facial treatment*

Sequential body toning systems

This is the term used to describe a new range of more sophisticated toning machines that are controlled by micro-processors.

Many combine iontophoresis, infra-red and programmed electro-stimulation over a frequency range of 100–800Hz. Session times will vary according to individual manufacturers and specific programmes, but on average treatment times are approximately 30–40 minutes. Infra-red is used to warm the area and thus improve the effectiveness of the treatment as current transmission will be maximised. Specialised products are applied to the area together with electrodes to release trapped fatty deposits while at the same time sequential electro-stimulation of the muscles, commencing at the ankles and gradually progressing upwards, increases the lymphatic and circulatory system to help in the dispersal of the accumulated waste products and the mobilised fat. Another key feature of such systems is that the programme can be adapted to meet the individual client's needs.

Treatments should be given in courses of approximately twelve over a one month period for optimum results with a regular maintenance programme thereafter.

Fig. 7.5 *Sequential body toning equipment*

224

POINT TO NOTE ▷ *Specific sequencing EMS units are specially designed to closely emulate exercise by varied passive stimulation and the range of frequency, 5–70 Hz, is controlled to stimulate most effectively the range of muscle fibre activity. These units use advanced micro processor control and offer a constantly changing parameter of stimulation. They follow the latest research into electrical muscular stimulation.*

Ultra-sound treatments

Treatment with ultra-sound has been in existence for a long time and is traditionally used by physiotherapists. It incorporates wave-type sound energy of a frequency which is just about audible which is transmitted via a flat, disk-shaped applicator to the tissues. It is able to penetrate to a depth of approximately 6 cm depending on the type of tissue. It agitates the cells, releasing toxins and fatty accumulations.

It is an effective treatment not only for muscular tensions, but also for cellulite and related disorders. A specialised coupling cream is normally used in conjunction with the treatment.

Interferential therapy

Interferential current is an alternative type of muscle stimulation to faradic that produces practically no sensation during treatment. The reason for this is that two medium frequency currents are delivered to the treatment area by separate circuits.

Where the two currents meet, a third frequency is produced. This is equivalent to the difference between the two original frequencies. There is no surge or interruption during treatment.

Interferential currents are used in therapy treatments for a number of reasons;

* A constant 'third frequency' will have an analgesic action which will help to reduce pain.
* A variable 'third frequency' will improve localised circulation, lymph drainage and cell metabolism which will help to reduce toxins and waste accumulations.

PROGRESS CHECK

1 What conditions are treated with specialised galvanic/high frequency/faradic treatments?
2 Give the main benefits of galvanic/high frequency facial treatments.
3 What systems of the body will be affected by a sequential body toning treatment?
4 Describe interferential current.

Specialised slimming programmes

Over the last few years manufacturers have been researching and developing slimming programmes incorporating a variety of heat, vibration, galvanic, faradic and specialised products. A typical treatment can involve;

- Detailed consultation with measurements being taken.
- Pressure massage.
- Heat therapy such as a sauna with the use of products that contain ingredients such as seaweed.
- Interrupted direct current on accupressure points (which may help to reduce appetite).
- The client is wrapped in polythene type sheeting which induces perspiration.
- Vibration and heat from the bed form the next stage of the treatment. The heat is normally derived from infra-red lamps.
- Finally the treatment finishes with a shower and measurements being checked and home care and retail advice given.

POINT TO NOTE ▷ *There are likely to be major developments in specialised slimming treatments over the coming years.*

Skin testers

Electronic skin testers for registering the pH of the skin are widely used in the Far East, and are gaining in popularity throughout the world.

Pressure massage

This is the name given to a range of specialist equipment which causes 'pneumatic' compression of the limbs. Pressure is delivered in a rhythmical manner thus simulating the natural pumping action of

Fig. 7.6 *The flux system of Press-o-therapy*

muscles and aiding lymphatic flow. The treatment primarily affects the vascular system so is excellent for helping many conditions associated with inefficient blood and lymph circulation, including gravitational oedema and the early stages of cellulite.

Treatment times will vary, but an average session will last about 20–30 minutes and can be combined with other salon services such as facials and massage.

ACTIVITY

Research manufacturers who offer the following:

a AHA treatments

b sequential body toning and specific sequencing EMS

c specialised high frequency/galvanic treatments

d body wraps

e micro-electrotherapy treatments.

KEY TERMS

You need to know what these words and phrases mean. Go back through the chapter to find out.

Cellulite treatments
Stretch mark treatments
Alpha Hydroxy Acids
Body wraps
Toning tables

Micro-electrotherapy
Specialised galvanic/high frequency/faradic/NMES treatments
Specialised slimming programmes
Pressure massage

8 Spa treatments

After working through this chapter you will be able to:
➤ identify the different types of spa treatment
➤ list the contraindications to spa treatments
➤ describe the effects of spa treatments
➤ understand the preparation required for a variety of spa treatments
➤ competently carry out a variety of spa treatments on clients.

Hydrotherapy

The therapeutic and social benefits of water have been used by all cultures for centuries. The Romans developed bath houses containing large hot and cool baths. People would progress from the coolest through to the hottest and finish, if they wished, with a cool plunge. Communal bathing was common practice in Roman society. There are only a few of the original Roman baths found today in the United Kingdom. The best and most famous examples are the Roman baths at Bath in England (hence the name 'Bath').

Health spas in European countries such as Austria and Germany have proved highly popular for years. The bathing in and drinking of mineral water along with additional treatment rooms have developed over the centuries and are often recommended by medical practitioners for their therapeutic benefits.

Health hydros and spas have increased rapidly in popularity over the past decade mainly due to the public's growing awareness of stress, health and personal appearance.

Today a common occurrence is for children to go to their local swimming baths with friends and for adults to attend health and leisure clubs for health and relaxation. If you asked a cross section of children through to adults to list three things they most enjoy on holiday you could be quite certain that the majority of people will include swimming in their list.

POINT TO NOTE ▷ *Hydrotherapy means treatment with water in any physical state (i.e. liquid, water vapour, steam, ice).*

Heat treatments

Heat treatments are used either as a spa treatment for relaxation or to prepare clients for further salon treatments such as massage. Over the last decade they have grown in popularity and can be found in local council sport centres, health and fitness clubs, health spas and in larger salons offering body treatments. There are a variety of different heat treatments which are continually being added to.

The general effects of heat treatments

1 Increase body temperature.

2 Metabolism is increased as heating of the body accelerates the natural chemical reactions that occur within the body, e.g. burning of energy, production of carbon dioxide. This in turn will increase the demand for oxygen and nutrients within the tissues, therefore increasing the amount of waste produced.

3 Circulation is increased. As the temperature in the body is increased the blood vessels dilate to allow the blood to flow more quickly to the surface thus reducing the body temperature. Other factors which trigger this process, known as vasodilation, are the stimulation of the sensory nerve endings and an increase in the body's metabolism.

4 Blood pressure is lowered as the pulse rate increases, causing the superficial blood vessels to dilate which automatically lowers the blood pressure due to the reduced resistance to the flow of blood through the blood vessels.

5 The heart rate increases to meet the demands of the body on the circulatory system.

6 Perspiration is induced to help cool the body, this aids removal of waste from the body and has a cleansing and softening effect on the skin.

7 The activity of the sudoriferous and sebaceous glands is increased.

8 Muscle fibres are relaxed in preparation for further salon treatment, e.g. massage.

9 Sensory nerve endings are soothed by mild heat.

10 A sense of general relaxation is achieved.

USEFUL INFORMATION

Hyperaemia is the term given to describe the increase in the flow of blood brought about by vasodilation.

POINT TO NOTE ▷ *The effects of heat treatments will vary according to the length and type of treatment given.*

General safety precautions to be observed in the spa area

* Ensure all equipment is serviced regularly.
* Always follow manufacturer's instructions.
* Hygiene is of the utmost importance, so ensure all equipment is maintained and cleaned according to the manufacturer's recommendations.

* Floors in the spa area should be non-slip.
* Spillages should be cleared up immediately.
* Clean towels and gowns must be regularly replenished.
* Dirty laundry baskets should be emptied regularly.
* Soaps, shampoos, body lotions should be replenished.
* Clients must always be checked for contraindications.

Sauna

In Scandinavian countries, pine log cabins were found by the side of lakes to enable people to take a cool dip in between sessions in the sauna. Today they are commonly found both indoors and outdoors. Saunas produce dry hot air and the pine logs absorb the condensation produced in the sauna.

A sauna resembles a wooden cabin, they are usually made from pine logs or panels which are packed together with insulating material (fibre glass) to prevent heat loss and ensure the heated air remains dry. They contain pine shelving at different heights for resting on. Pine slats (duck boards) on the floor protect clients' feet from heated flooring which could burn them. A thermostatically controlled electric stove is used to heat the sauna on top of which is a tray of non-splintering stones (coals). Manufacturers should ensure that the heating capacity of the electric stoves have the correct power rating for the size of the sauna.

When installing saunas the contractors should check that there is sufficient space around the cabin to enable air to circulate. An air inlet is found at floor level and an outlet is found near the top of the cabin. As the power rating for sauna stoves is much higher than for normal household electrical appliances, the sauna stove is fitted directly to the consumer's mains electrical supply. (They cannot be run from a plug socket !) A thermometer should be placed as near as possible to the roof of the sauna to accurately measure the temperature inside the sauna. It is important to have some way for a client to measure time whilst in a sauna so either an egg timer or clock should be in the sauna or a clock on a wall outside which can be seen through the window of the sauna door.

Note. Remember to make sure timers are working correctly.

Fig. 8.1 *Sauna stove*

Water can be ladled onto the coals of the sauna stove. This creates steam and increases the humidity in the sauna, which in turn reduces the rate of the evaporation of sweat from the client's skin making the sauna feel hotter. Hot air does not have the same heat capacity as hot water, therefore the temperature of a sauna does not feel as hot on the skin as water would. The temperature of a sauna can vary between 50–120°C (the boiling point of water is 100°C).

POINTS TO NOTE ▷
* *If the air is too dry the body's natural perspiration evaporates quickly, which has a cooling effect on the skin, and signs of dehydration such as tiredness and dry throats can occur.*
* *If the humidity of the air is too high, perspiration produced to assist in the cooling of the body does not evaporate leaving people feeling hot and clammy.*
* *A hygrometer is used to measure humidity.*

GOOD PRACTICE ▷
* *A comfortable sauna temperature for a new client unaccustomed to a sauna treatment is 60–80°C.*
* *A comfortable sauna humidity is approximately 50–60%.*
* *As hot air rises, a thermometer should be placed near the top of the sauna.*

Care of the sauna

1 Hygiene is of utmost importance as although the air in the sauna is too hot for growth of micro organisms, bacterial infection could be housed and grow in the wooden walls and furnishings of the sauna due to the warm, moist conditions.

2 The sauna should be regularly disinfected by scrubbing the benches and floor with disinfectant products recommended by the manufacturer.

3 Disposable client footwear can be used to reduce the risk of passing contagious foot conditions such as verrucas.

4 At the end of the day, the sauna doors should be left open to allow for a change of air. This prevents stale odours from lingering.

CONTRAINDICATIONS   to a sauna

! Low and high blood pressure.

! Heart conditions.

! Thrombosis or phlebitis.

! Bronchitis.

! Asthma.

USEFUL INFORMATION

The moisture content of the air is referred to as humidity. Relative humidity is the measurement of moisture content as a percentage of the maximum it can hold at that temperature. 100% is the maximum capacity of moisture content in air.

60–70% relative humidity is a comfortable humidity for working conditions.

As the temperature of air increases, so does its capacity for holding moisture, e.g. if the temperature of a salon was 20°C and the relative humidity measurement was 70%, then raising the room temperature to 100°C would decrease the relative humidity to approximately 20%.

The relative humidity in a sauna can be as low as 10%. This causes perspiration to evaporate very quickly, thus causing a cooling effect on the skin so that the sauna does not feel as hot as the actual temperature recorded in the sauna. Water loss is from the whole of the body and it should be remembered that if the temperature is high and the relative humidity is low then there is a danger of dehydration, breathing difficulties and scorching of the lungs.

! Epilepsy.

! Dysfunction of the nervous system.

! Oedema.

! Recent scar tissue.

! Severe bruising.

! Diabetes.*

! Early stages of menstruation.

! Pregnancy.*

! Heavy colds/fever.

! Infectious skin diseases.

! Athletes foot.

! Verrucas.

! Sunburn.

! Claustrophobia.

! After alcohol consumption.

! After a heavy meal.

* Only to be carried out with medical approval.

Effects of a sauna

* Increases body temperature.
* Metabolism is increased.
* Blood pressure is lowered.
* Pulse rate increases.
* Circulation increases.
* Perspiration is induced which aids removal of waste from the body and has a cleansing and softening effect on the skin.
* The activity of the sudoriferous and sebaceous glands is increased.
* Muscle fibres are relaxed in preparation for further salon treatment, e.g. massage.
* A sense of well being is achieved.

Preparation of the sauna

1 Observe general safety precautions.

2 The sauna stove is switched on to allow the temperature of the sauna to build up prior to use. A large sauna will take approximately one hour to heat up where as a smaller sauna will take approximately thirty minutes.

3 The air vents should be open to allow the air to circulate.

4 A pine bucket filled with water is placed in the sauna with a ladle. Pine fragrance can be added to the water to produce a pleasant fresh smell when used on the coals.

5 Paper towels may be placed on the floor.

6 Showers are checked and appropriate products are made available for clients, e.g. shower gels and caps.

7 Towels are replenished.

8 Throughout the day the laundry basket is emptied and towels, etc. replenished

Note. Different establishments will offer different services to clients and will outline these to therapists in their induction programme, e.g. towels may be placed in the sauna for clients to rest on, clean bath robes may be placed in the sauna area.

GOOD PRACTICE ▷ *The overall hygiene of the spa reflects on everyone working there so it is paramount that a therapist uses their initiative to refill products, empty laundry baskets, replenish towels and clean areas as needed – **don't** wait to be asked. Ensuring the work place is kept clean and tidy is part of a therapist's job.*

Sauna treatment

1 Client is greeted at reception and taken to a changing area.

2 Consultation is carried out to check for contraindications and to explain effects of treatment.

Note. In health spas a detailed consultation is undertaken on the guest's arrival by a member of their medical staff. The therapists would still explain the effects of the treatment to a new guest.

3 Client removes items such as contact lenses, glasses and jewellery before showering to remove deodorants, body lotions, fragrances, etc.

4 Client is taken to sauna and advised if it is their first treatment to spend approximately 5–8 minutes on a lower shelf, allowing them time to adjust to the temperature of the sauna. It must be stressed to the client that if at any time they feel light-headed they must come out of the sauna.

5 Therapist informs client of the time and asks them to take a cool shower or use the plunge pool for a short time to cool the body, stop perspiration and tighten the pores which have dilated due to the heat of the sauna and through perspiration. The temperature of the plunge pool/shower should be approximately 15–21°C.

6 The client can return to the sauna for 10–20 minute periods in between taking cool showers or using the plunge pool for up to a total treatment time of approximately 30 minutes.

7 The client should relax after a sauna either in a rest area or by having a further treatment such as a massage and drink plenty of fluids to prevent dehydration.

POINT TO NOTE ▷ *Male clients tend to prefer a higher sauna temperature to females.*

GOOD PRACTICE ▷ *Time is money so ensure treatment times are observed. Don't be tempted if you have some free time to allow clients to spend longer in the sauna as next time they will think you are giving them less for the same price!*

ACTIVITY	Research the different size saunas available, noting their client capacity, initial setting up and running costs. Evaluate which would prove to be the most cost effective for a large salon, hotel and health spa.

Vibratory sauna

The vibratory sauna machine looks like an elongated steam cabinet as it allows a client to lie flat inside it. It is manufactured from moulded plastic with a vibrating couch which has a built-in head rest. Control panels on the outside allow the therapist to set the temperature, duration, vibration along with the stereo and fan control for cooling the sauna. There are control panels situated at a convenient location inside the chamber to enable the client to alter the temperature, music and to operate the fan. During treatment heat is introduced into the sauna whilst the couch vibrates gently, to relax the client's muscles and help reduce stress. The built-in stereo system allows the therapist to play therapeutic tapes and aromatic oils can be used to further enhance the client's relaxation.

USEFUL INFORMATION

Skin can tolerate much higher air temperatures than water temperatures.

Fig. 8.2 *A vibratory sauna*

CONTRAINDICATIONS to vibratory saunas

- ! Thrombosis or phlebitis.
- ! Circulatory conditions.
- ! Infectious skin conditions.
- ! Sunburn.
- ! Pregnancy.*
- ! Menstruation.
- ! Heavy colds or fevers.
- ! After alcohol or a heavy meal.
- ! Low and high blood pressure.
- ! Epilepsy.
- ! Diabetes.*
- ! Dysfunction of the nervous system.
- ! Oedema.
- ! Recent scar tissue.
- ! Athletes foot.
- ! Verrucas.

* Only to be carried out with medical approval.

POINT TO NOTE ▷ *The vibratory sauna is a personal treatment, the temperature can be set to suit the individual client.*

Effects of a vibratory sauna

- Increases body temperature.
- Increases circulation.
- Heart rate increases.
- Pulse rate increases.
- Blood pressure is lowered.
- Increases metabolism.
- Induces perspiration.
- Relaxes muscle fibres.

Care of the vibratory sauna

The sauna should be cleaned between clients according to the manufacturer's instructions.

Preparation of the vibratory sauna

1 General safety precautions should be observed.

2 Fresh paper towels are placed over the vibratory couch.

3 The sauna should be switched on at the mains. (There is no need to preheat the chamber.)

Vibratory sauna treatment

1 Client is greeted at reception and taken to a changing area.

2 Consultation is carried out to check for contraindications and to explain the effects of the treatment.

3 Client removes items such as glasses and jewellery prior to showering to remove deodorants, fragrances, body lotions, etc.

4 The client is helped into the cabinet and the therapist switches on the vibratory couch and music.

5 The room lights may be dimmed or the client may opt to wear eye shields.

6 At the end of the treatment, the body is cooled slightly by the fans which automatically cut in.

7 The client is helped out of the cabinet and may take a cool shower prior to resting. The drinking of suitable fluids is recommended.

GOOD PRACTICE ▷

- *Some clients are irritated by music so therapeutic tapes should only be used with the client's agreement.*
- *As clients are all individuals, it is important to establish what types of fragrance they like before selecting aromatic oils.*

PROGRESS CHECK

1 Define hydrotherapy.

2 List the ten general effects of heat treatments.

3 Explain the term 'relative humidity' and its relevance to a sauna treatment.

4 Give four points that should be considered when taking care of the sauna.

5 Describe in detail the preparation, client consultation, treatment and after care advice given for a sauna treatment.

6 State the effects of a vibratory sauna treatment. Also state four contraindications to treatment.

Steam treatments

Steam treatments were first used by the Turks or Romans and are sometimes referred to as a Turkish bath. The original Turkish or Roman baths were found in large buildings which contained steam baths of various temperatures, where people met socially for a relaxing bath.

There are two main types of steam treatment available, steam rooms/ cabinets or steam baths. Both enable clients to receive a 'wet heat' or 'moist heat' treatment.

Steam cabinets

Steam cabinets are designed for individual treatment enabling clients to sit in the cabinet with their heads outside so that they can breathe in the normal air of the room.

A modern steam cabinet can be constructed from either metal or moulded fibreglass. The fibreglass model is more expensive but is easier to clean and as less towels are needed to protect the client from the heat of the metal they tend to be more popular, even though they tend to be more expensive.

Steam cabinets have an opening for the client's head and a hinged door for easy access to and from the cabinet making them more suitable than saunas for clients who have a tendency to suffer from claustrophobia. Inside there is an adjustable seat which is raised or lowered according to the client's height. Beneath the seat at floor level is a water tank, made from cast iron or aluminium, which is heated by an electrical element. The size of the water tank varies and should be considered when purchasing a steam cabinet. The larger the capacity of the tank the longer it can be used before the therapist needs to refill it. Therefore in a spa where the steam cabinets receive more use, a cabinet with a large water tank would be more beneficial.

To operate the steam cabinet the therapist will find a:

- Mains switch on the wall. The cabinet must be fitted direct to the mains electrical supply due to the power rating of the heating element.
- Timer switch to set the time for prior heating of the cabinet and the actual treatment time.
- Temperature gauge to set the cabinet to the appropriate temperature.

Fig. 8.3 *Steam cabinet*

237

The timer and the temperature gauge are generally found adjacent to each other on the outside of the cabinet often at floor level near the heating element.

Steam cabinets produce wet heat as the thermostatically controlled water tank heats the water until it boils producing wet steam which mixes with the air inside the cabinet or room creating water vapour (at a lower temperature than the 100°C required to boil water) at a temperature tolerable to the skin. The highest temperature advised for use in a steam treatment for the body is 45°C.

The relative humidity of the air inside the steam cabinet or bath is generally around 92–97%. As the air is virtually saturated the sweat produced by the sudoriferous glands, due to the heating of the body by the water vapour, is unable to evaporate and cool the body and therefore it trickles off the body.

POINT TO NOTE ▷ *The body will replace any lost fluids during a heat treatment. It will absorb extra water from the intestines which can lead to constipation or create further problems for those clients who suffer with this condition.*

Steam rooms

Steam rooms accommodate a number of clients who may take a treatment at the same time. This type of treatment is becoming more popular in Europe where social attitudes to exposed bodies are far less puritanical than in, say, Far Eastern countries where body treatments are only just beginning to increase in popularity.

The length of time for a steam room to heat up ready for use will depend upon its size. Some are designed for individual use whilst others can accommodate up to eight people. Individual steam 'tubes' provide a mini-steam-room environment which takes up a small amount of space and is easily affordable for salons.

Advantages of using a steam cabinet

For the client:

- Steam cabinets are a more private treatment than the communal steam room.
- The temperature can be adjusted to suit the individual client.
- Clients are able to keep their head out and keep their hair dry.
- It is far more suitable for claustrophobic clients as their head is out of the steam.
- The client is able to breathe in the air in the room rather than steam.

For the salon:

- The running costs are much lower than with a steam room as the heating element in a steam cabinet uses far less power.

USEFUL INFORMATION

Breathing in hot air of a high relative humidity can cause water-logging of the lungs as the air is cooled and water condensed from it as it enters the body.

238

* The initial financial outlay is much lower.
* The space required to accommodate the cabinet in the salon is much smaller.

Care of steam cabinets and rooms

1 Hygiene is extremely important as moist heat provides an ideal breeding environment for micro-organisms.

2 The steam baths and rooms must be cleaned down with suitable disinfectants recommended by the manufacturers before and after treatment.

3 The doors of the steam bath and room should be left open at the end of the day to allow for an interchange of fresh air, preventing stale odours.

4 Disposable footwear can be used to prevent the risk of cross-infection of contagious foot conditions.

CONTRAINDICATIONS to steam treatments for the body

! Thrombosis or phlebitis.

! Asthma and other respiratory conditions.

! Low or high blood pressure.

! Heart conditions.

! Epilepsy.

! Diabetes.*

! Athletes foot.

! Verrucas.

! Infectious skin diseases.

! Sunburn.

! Pregnancy.*

! Menstruation.

! Clients on restricted diets who may have a tendency to become light-headed.

! Heavy colds/fevers.

! After a heavy meal or alcohol.

! Claustrophobia.**

! Dysfunction of the nervous system.

! Severe bruising.

! Recent scar tissue.

*   Only to be carried out with medical approval.
** Some clients find the steam cabinet less claustrophobic.

239

POINT TO NOTE ▷ *If given approval by a medical practitioner, clients with skin conditions such as psoriasis and eczema may receive wet heat treatments as they may help these conditions.*

Effects of a steam treatment for the body

* Body temperature rises.
* Metabolism is increased.
* Circulation is increased.
* Heart rate increases.
* Pulse rate increases.
* Blood pressure is lowered.
* Perspiration is induced.
* Cleansing and softening of the skin.
* Superficial muscles are relaxed.

Preparation of the steam cabinet

1 Observe general safety precautions.

2 The cabinet is cleaned with sterilising liquid.

3 Metal heating trough is filled with water.

4 Towel is placed over seat to protect the client and if using a metal bath, towels must be placed inside to protect the client. Place a towel over the opening in the bath to prevent heat loss.

5 The water tank guard must be in place so as to protect the client from burning themselves.

6 Turn on the mains switch and set the temperature gauge to maximum to heat the bath. Set the timer to allow sufficient time for the bath to heat. (This will vary depending on the capacity of the water tank. Note the manufacturer's recommendations for heating time. A general guide for the time taken for a small tank to heat is approximately 15 minutes.)

7 Once heated, adjust the temperature gauge to 50–55°C and check the timer switch does not click off allowing the temperature to fall.

Steam cabinet treatment

1 Greet client at reception and take them to changing facilities.

2 Consultation is carried out to check for contraindications and to explain the treatment and its effects.

3 Client removes items such as jewellery, glasses and contact lenses and showers to remove deodorants, fragrances, body lotions, etc.

4 The client is helped into the bath. A fresh towel is placed around the client's neck for protection and to prevent heat loss.

5 The timer is set to the appropriate time, generally 15–20 minutes.

6 The therapist should reassure the client throughout the treatment and be at hand should they need them.

7 At the end of the treatment, help the client from the bath and direct them into a cool shower.

8 The use of an exfoliating product is recommended to speed up cellular regeneration and general skin texture.

9 The client should relax after the steam treatment and drink plenty of liquids.

GOOD PRACTICE ▷ *It is important to look directly at the client's face and not at the client's body when helping them in and out of baths and showers. Imagine how you would feel if a fully clothed person stared at your naked body!*

ACTIVITY

With a colleague, design and carry out a survey to establish the percentage of people in your local area who have undertaken a heat treatment in the last twelve months. Note the type of treatment, the age ranges, gender and reasons for treatment.

Floatation treatments

There are two types of floatation treatment; *wet floatation* and *dry floatation*.

Wet floatation tank

These are made from moulded fibreglass and can vary in size. They are generally rectangular, shaped like a small room, with a door opening outwards on the side of the tank. Inside the interior colour is usually blue and there is approximately 12 inches of warm, saturated salt water heated to body temperature on the floor surface, which will allow everyone to float. A small interior light illuminates the tank enabling the client time to climb in and settle before switching it off. The switch control is in easy reach on the side wall.

The tanks are often found in health spas and leisure centres and are situated in a separate room with access to a shower. Clients are advised to shower to remove any body creams, etc., and to apply petroleum jelly to any cuts preventing the brine (salt water) from entering any abrasions and causing a stinging sensation. It is suggested that no clothing is worn in the tank. Ear plugs are provided and often a neck cushion, which can be very reassuring to the weak or non-swimmer who believes they cannot float. A small step at the side of the tank allows the client to climb easily into the illuminated tank and a pull bar allows easy closure of the door. The client can take their time to adjust to the warm, slightly restrictive environment before switching off the interior light. There is usually an intercom system which enables the therapist to check the client is comfortable, play therapeutic music and reassures the apprehensive client that someone is at hand should they need them. The tanks generally have a small, round ventilation hole which also allows the client to be phased into total darkness by first switching off the interior light and using a delay switch to turn the lighting off in the outer room (light can still enter the tank from the outer room through the door frame and the ventilation hole). This is extremely beneficial for apprehensive clients. The client lies on their back, the neck supported if they wish by a neck cushion, allowing the brine water to support their body thus relaxing all superficial muscles and releasing tension in the body. If the client wishes, therapeutic background music is played and after the client has had sufficient time to drift off, the music quietly ends allowing a peaceful and tranquil period before the music is quietly reintroduced, slowly bringing the treatment to an end.

Afterwards the client needs to shower to remove the brine from their skin and hair using professional products that could also be sold to them by the therapist.

Health spas book an hour treatment. Out of this the client would spend 40–45 minutes in the floatation tank.

After a beneficial treatment the exhilarating, uplifting experience of 'walking on air' brought about by the total relaxation of mind and body can make this an almost addictive treatment.

Care of the floatation tank

1 The tank must be free of debris such as oils, scum, loose hairs, etc.

2 The inside of the tank, above the water line, must be cleaned a minimum of once a week or as necessary.

3 The water in the tank must be filtered between uses and the temperature checked.

4 The level of the water has to be checked between clients.

Fig. 8.4 *Wet floatation*

5 The pH of the water should be 7.6. This should be checked on a daily basis.

6 The level of bromine must not be higher than 2 p.p.m. and must be checked a minimum of once a week.

7 The tank must be tested either by an independent laboratory or by the Environmental Health Department.

CONTRAINDICATIONS

to wet floatation

! Claustrophobia.

! Highly nervous clients.

! Severe cuts/abrasions.

! Recent scar tissue.

! Infectious skin diseases.

! Severe eczema/psoriasis.

! Plantar wart (verruca).

! Tinea pedis (athletes foot).

! After alcohol consumption.

! Heart conditions.*

! Epilepsy.*

! After a heavy meal.

* Only to be carried out with medical approval.

Effects of a wet floatation treatment
* Warms the body tissues aiding relaxation.
* Relaxes muscles through the buoyancy of the water.
* Eases aches and pains.
* A general feeling of well being is achieved.

Preparation of the wet floatation tank

1 Observe general safety precautions.

2 Check the tank and shower areas are clean.

3 Ensure the level and temperature of the water are correct.

Wet floatation treatment

1 Greet client at reception and take them to changing facilities.

2 Consultation is carried out to check for contraindications and to explain the effects of the treatment.

3 Client removes items such as jewellery, glasses, etc., and may shower.

243

4 Client protects any minor skin abrasions with petroleum jelly and inserts ear plugs.

5 Client enters floatation tank, closes door and in their own time switches off the interior light.

6 If the client wishes, the therapist can play piped music during the floatation time.

7 At the end of the treatment the therapist would advise the client to shower to remove the salt from skin and hair.

8 The client should rest in a relaxation room and drink fluids as required.

Dry floatation tank

Dry floatation tanks were originally developed in Austria and have been extremely popular there for many years. They are made of a stainless steel frame containing a tank of water which can be thermostatically controlled, into which a duck board is set which can be lowered to suspend the client in water with no pressure points. The water tank is sealed by a flexible membrane, the tank is clad in upholstered panels which make it appear rectangular in shape, similar to a bath tub.

The client lies on the raised bench which is protected by paper roll. Protective paper sheeting may be placed over them. The therapist pushes a control button to lower the board thus suspending the client's body weight, protected by vinyl, in warm water, the temperature of which remains constant.

The dry tanks are mainly found in health spas in treatment rooms with easy access to a shower. The dry floatation method can be used in a number of treatments some of which involve coating the body in various ingredients for different effects, e.g. mud can be used for its exfoliating and softening effects, a mixture of hay softened with its own juices and eucalyptus essential oil is said to be beneficial for sluggish lymph circulation and respiratory conditions and milk and essential oils can be used for softening the skin and has therapeutic benefits. The floatation can be given on its own for the therapeutic benefit of releasing tension in the body and for relaxation.

Once the client is suspended in the dry floatation tank the therapist switches on gentle therapeutic music, dims the lights and places an alert button within easy reach of the client. The client is then left to relax for approximately 40 minutes.

The therapist will check on the client's comfort after 5–8 minutes, remaining close at hand outside the door throughout the duration of the treatment and returning to the room at the end. The control button is pressed which slowly raises the board under the client's back and brings them back to the top of the tank, the vinyl cover is removed and the client is helped off. If a specific treatment such as mud has been used the therapist will have to place protective covering on the floor between the tank and the shower.

Care of the dry floatation tank
The tank should be cleaned with a sterilising liquid recommended by the manufacturer.

CONTRAINDICATIONS to dry floatation

! Infectious skin conditions.

! Severe respiratory conditions.

! Heavy colds/fevers.

! Heart conditions.*

! Diabetes.*

! Epilepsy.*

* Only to be carried out with medical approval.

Effects of a dry floatation treatment
* Aids relaxation.
* Relaxes muscles through the buoyancy effect of the water.
* Eases aches and pains.
* A general sense of well being is achieved.

Note. If specific treatments are used in conjunction with dry floatation then the specific benefits from these can be added to the above list.

Preparation for a dry floatation treatment
1 Observe general safety precautions.

2 The vinyl sheeting must be clean, dry and protected as necessary.

3 The board is raised to the top of the tank and the temperature control switch is turned to pre-heat the water.

Dry floatation treatment
1 Greet client at reception and take them to changing facilities.

2 Consultation is carried out to check for contraindications and to explain the effects of the treatment.

3 Client removes items such as jewellery, glasses, etc., and may shower.

4 The client lies on top of the tank and the therapist covers them.

5 The therapist presses a switch which lowers the board.

6 The lights are dimmed and music played to suit the individual client.

7 At the end of the floatation time the therapist raises the board and helps the client up.

8 If specific treatments such as mud baths have been given, the client showers to remove the products from their body.

9 The client should relax in a rest room and drink fluids as needed.

PROGRESS CHECK

1 List four contraindications for each of the following treatments:
  a steam cabinet
  b wet floatation
  c dry floatation.

2 For each of the following treatments describe two effects:
  a steam room
  b wet floatation.

3 Describe how a steam cabinet operates.

4 State the advantages for the client and salon of using a steam cabinet.

5 Explain the preparation, consultation, treatment and after care advice given for a dry floatation treatment.

Foam baths

Foam baths are far more likely to be found in a health hydro offering a variety of spa treatments than in a beauty salon where the costs of purchase, installation and running could prove too high an expense. However modifications to a general household bath can transform it for use as a foam bath.

Foam baths found in health hydros are found in the spa area and resemble a household bath in appearance. A perforated, plastic duck board is found at the bottom of the bath which will allow compressed air to be forced through the hundreds of tiny holes into the bath water. Only a small quantity of water is needed, approximately 10–15 cm to cover the duck board. The water is heated to between 37–43°C depending on the individual client. Concentrated foam essence such as seaweed is added to the water prior to the compressor being switched on. The compressor pumps air to beneath the duck board where it will force its way through the perforated holes to aerate the water. The compressor is left on until the foam created by the aeration of the water and foam essence reaches the top of the bath. The client lies in the foam in a semi-reclined position with their head resting on the back of the bath, outside of the foam.

USEFUL INFORMATION

Body heat is retained in a foam bath as detergent foam acts as an insulator, so the heat in the client's body cannot escape. The heat will increase, inducing perspiration and giving the client the general benefits of raising the body temperature. (This is unlike a normal bath where the temperature of the water and body fall quite quickly unless hot water is continually added.)

Fig. 8.5 *Foam bath*

POINT TO NOTE $\rhd$ *Foam is made up of approximately 10% water and 90% air.*

Care of the foam bath

The bath should be cleaned between client use with a sterilising fluid recommended by the manufacturer.

CONTRAINDICATIONS to foam baths

! Infectious skin conditions.

! Verrucas.

! Athletes foot.

! Sunburn.

! After consuming alcohol.

! Diabetes.*

! Epileptics.*

! Respiratory conditions.*

! Circulatory conditions.*

* Only to be carried out with medical approval.

Effects of a foam bath

* Induces perspiration.
* Raises body temperature.
* Induces circulation.
* Muscle fibres are relaxed.

Preparation of the foam bath

1 The bath is cleaned and filled with sufficient warm water to cover the duck board.

2 A selected concentrated foam essence is added to the water, e.g. seaweed.

3 The compressor is switched on to aerate the water.

4 Once the foam reaches the top of the bath the compressor is switched off. The foam bath is now ready for use.

Foam bath treatment

1 Client is greeted at reception and taken to changing facilities.

2 Consultation is carried out to check for contraindications and to explain the effects of the treatment.

3 Client removes items such as contact lenses, glasses and jewellery prior to showering to remove fragrances, deodorants, body lotions, etc.

4 Client is helped into the bath.

5 Treatment time is generally around 15 minutes.

6 Client is helped from the bath.

7 A warm shower may be taken using exfoliating products for cellular regeneration.

8 The client should relax in a rest area and drink fluids as required.

Aerated baths

There are many types of aerated bath to be found in health spas, hydros and clubs, and they can also be found in hotels and individual homes. They vary in size, shape and price. The simplest form is a normal household bath with an air pump outside which pumps air into the water.

Aerated baths were developed in France. They are filled with water and air is forced into the water either through a hose or through holes in a duck board in the bath. Essence may be added to aerated baths for their individual properties. Treatment time would last approximately 15 minutes.

Hydrotherapy bath

Aerated baths are used as a hydrotherapy treatment in the majority of health spas, using a hose to direct air over the body. The hydrotherapy unit is shaped like a bath with grab handles to assist the client to get in and out. The inside of the hydrotherapy unit is fitted to the shape of the client's body more so than an ordinary household bath. The unit is filled with warm water, the selected essence is added and the compressor is switched on allowing air to aerate the bath gently through the duck board. The client is helped into the bath and the therapist switches on the hose which is worked methodically over the muscle groups. The treatment time is generally around 20 minutes.

Fig. 8.6 *Hydrotherapy bath*

ACTIVITY	Research the range of hydrotherapy units available and compare their benefits and cost.

CONTRAINDICATIONS to hydrotherapy baths

! Heart conditions.

! Infectious skin conditions.

! Circulatory conditions.

! After a heavy meal or after consuming alcohol.

! Athletes foot.

! Verrucas.

! Pregnancy.

! Diabetes.*

! Epilepsy.*

* Only to be carried out with medical approval.

Effects of a hydrotherapy bath

* Body temperature is raised.
* Perspiration is induced.
* Circulation is increased.
* Muscle fibres are relaxed.
* Metabolism is increased.

Preparation of the hydrotherapy bath

1 Observe general safety precautions.

2 Fill bath with warm water.

3 Add essence required.

Hydrotherapy treatment

1 Client is greeted at reception and taken to changing facilities.

2 Consultation is carried out and the effects of the treatment are explained.

3 Client removes items such as glasses, jewellery, etc., and showers to remove deodorant, fragrances, body lotions, etc.

4 Compressor is switched on for gentle aeration of the water.

5 The client is helped into the unit, where they rest in a semi-reclined position.

6 The hose is switched on and the therapist guides it over the client's body for approximately 15–20 minutes before the hose is switched off.

HEALTH AND BEAUTY THERAPY

7 The compressor is switched off and after a few minutes the client is helped from the bath.

8 The client is taken to a relaxation area to rest.

Whirlpools

Whirlpools are sometimes called spa baths and are commonly known by the name of the American manufacturer who brought them to commercial success – Jacuzzi™. They are found in the majority of health spas, hydros, clubs and hotels and even in individual homes. They vary in size, shape and price. The larger ones can accommodate up to eight people at the same time. They are commonly found near the swimming pool in most health spas where the benefits of contrast baths can be achieved.

There are a number of factors to consider when fitting a whirlpool:
1 The floor must be:
   * reinforced to take the large weight of the filled pool
   * tanked and drained.

2 The plant room which houses the controls must:
   * have a suitable power supply
   * be within five metres of the pool
   * be well ventilated.

3 The pool should have:
   * a filtration system
   * a heavy duty control panel to withstand constant wear and tear.

Research:

a the range of spa pools available

b the recommended chemical additives and how they are added, e.g. automatically or manually

c the manufacturers' procedures for checking the water quality and filters

d the manufacturers' procedures for maintaining the pH and ensuring hygienic practices.

Compare your findings to the SPATA code of practice.

Effects of the whirlpool

* Increases circulation.
* Stimulates the skin and aids desquamation.
* Increases metabolism.
* Relaxes muscles.
* Relieves aches and pains (whilst in pool).
* Produces a sense of well being.

Fig. 8.7 *Whirlpool bath*

The whirlpool generally has two massage effects; a gentle effect and a strong one. The gentle massage effect is created by compressed air flowing through small holes at the base of the pool. The strong whirlpool massage effect is created by jets of air pummelling the skin along with the action of the fast moving water of the pool. When these two effects are combined they create a fast stream of bubbling water.

ACTIVITY

With a colleague, select three different spa treatments that would benefit each of you. Taking the roles of client and therapist undertake the treatments selected and evaluate their physiological and psychological effects on you. Discuss and compare your findings with your colleague.

Hydro-oxygen baths

This treatment involves the client reclining in a bath-type cabinet which contains jets which are used to blast the client's body with hot water and to diffuse oxygen into the cabinet. The treatment is extremely stimulating and makes the skin more sensitive. An infra-red treatment would not follow due to skin sensitivity.

Fig. 8.8 *Hydro-oxygen bath*

POINT TO NOTE ⊳ *The temperature of the surface of the skin is 33°C or below.*

- *Water of a temperature above the skin's surface temperature has a hyper-thermal effect as it adds heat to the body.*
- *Water of a temperature below the skin's surface temperature has a hypo-thermal effect as it draws heat away from the body.*
- *When water is used to cool or warm the body it is referred to as hydrothermal therapy.*
- *When the mechanical properties of water, such as buoyancy, are used it is referred to as hydrokinetic therapy.*

Effects of hydrotherapy treatments

Hot baths:
- Relieve pain.
- Induce perspiration.
- Have a cleansing effect.
- Increase temperature.

Cold baths:
- Relieve pain.
- Have a stimulating effect.
- Have a diuretic effect.
- Reduce temperature.

USEFUL INFORMATION

The temperature of the surface of hands and feet is generally much lower than the temperature of the surface of the skin of the body (i.e. below 20°C).

Cold baths used to be very popular, particularly after a sauna. However clients today tend to prefer cool baths. Perhaps tolerance of different temperatures has altered with the advances in technology which brought about such developments as central heating and air conditioning.

GOOD PRACTICE ⊳ *The temperature in a therapeutic cold bath would be between 10–27°C.*

POINT TO NOTE ⊳ *The general effect of a cold bath is stimulating.*

Contrast baths

Contrast baths describe the situation where two different temperature baths are found next to each other so that the client can move from one to the other. The treatment time may vary slightly dependent on the temperature of the baths, but generally the client would spend between 1–5 minutes in the hot bath and 15–60 seconds in the cool bath. The total treatment time would last approximately 10–30 minutes.

The Scotch Douche treatment utilises hot and cold water which is alternatively run up and down the client's spine to stimulate the spinal nerves by sluicing blood in and out of the spinal area. This treatment is believed to help sufferers of migraines and other ailments such as aches and pains in the back.

The Sitz bath from Germany also uses the effects of contrast bathing in its treatment. Two baths are used, one containing hot water the other cold. For the first 5–10 minutes the client sits in the hot bath with their feet immersed in cold water. The client then changes and sits in the cold bath with their feet immersed in the hot water. The cold water causes the blood vessels to constrict which in turn will force the blood supply to the area of the body immersed in hot water. The overall effect of this treatment is to flush the blood into the pelvic area bringing nourishment to it then to flush it out taking away waste. This type of bath was recommended for any illness which effects the lower part of the body.

Another treatment using the effects of differing temperatures is the Spanish Mantle treatment. Cold, damp, cotton sheets are wrapped around the client and hot water bottles are placed around the body or a radiant heat lamp is used to induce perspiration. The client would be left to perspire for up to three hours. It was claimed that when the sheets were finally removed the elimination of toxins from the body changed the colouring of the sheets.

ACTIVITY

Research the different spa treatments offered by three different health spas.

PROGRESS CHECK

1 State the different treatments you might find in a spa area.
2 List four contraindications to each of the following treatments:
   a foam bath
   b hydrotherapy bath.
3 State two effects for each of the following treatments:
   a foam bath
   b hydrotherapy bath
   c whirlpool.
4 Explain the preparation of the foam bath.
5 State the effects of hydrotherapy treatments.
6 Briefly describe the following treatments:
   a hydro-oxygen baths
   b contrast baths.

KEY TERMS

You need to know what these words and phrases mean. Go back through the chapter to find out.

Hydrotherapy	Floatation treatments	Hydrotherapy bath
Heat treatments	Foam baths	Whirlpool
Sauna	Aerated baths	Hydro-oxygen baths
Steam cabinets/rooms		

9 Light therapy treatments

After working through this chapter you will be able to:
➤ outline the key principles of the electromagnetic spectrum
➤ state the differences between ultra-violet and infra-red treatments
➤ list the three bands of ultra-violet rays and explain their main effects
➤ give the main benefits and uses of infra-red and ultra-violet treatments
➤ list the contraindications and safety precautions to both treatments.

There are two main forms of radiation that the therapist needs to be aware of, each forming part of the electromagnetic spectrum. *Ultra-violet* is used mainly for its skin tanning effects while *infra-red* is used as a method of warming the tissues for therapeutic purposes.

The electromagnetic spectrum

The electromagnetic spectrum consists of a continuous band of radiation given off from the sun in varying frequencies and wavelengths. The radiation given off can be divided into bands according to their wavelength:

* Gamma rays (shortest wavelength).
* X-rays.
* Ultra-violet rays.
* Visible light (red, orange, yellow, green, blue, indigo, violet).
* Infra-red rays.
* Radio waves (longest wavelength).

Wavelengths are typically measured in nanometres (nm). A nanometre is a millionth of a millimetre. The wavelengths of visible light are in the range between 400 and 770 nm with the lower (shorter) wavelengths being at the blue end of the visible spectrum and the higher (longer) wavelengths being at the red end of the visible spectrum. Infra-red rays have wavelengths in the range of 770 to 4000 nm while ultra-violet rays have wavelengths between 200 to 400 nm.

Electromagnetic rays can be uniquely defined in terms of their wavelength. The wavelength is defined as the distance from the point on one wave to the same point on the next wave. Rays also have a frequency which is defined as the number of cycles or complete waves that pass a fixed point each second. Frequency is calculated and shown as a reading of Hertz, i.e. the number of cycles per second. Shorter wavelengths such as ultra-violet will have a higher frequency than longer wavelengths such as infra-red because they require more cycles to cover the same distance.

Fig. 9.1 *The electromagnetic spectrum*

254

The bands of radiation used in therapy treatments are ultra-violet and infra-red.

Infra-red radiation

As mentioned previously, infra-red rays have wavelengths of the order 770 to 4000 nm which means that they have longer wavelengths than visible light. This form of radiation can be divided into two bands:

* Infra-red rays which are longer wavelength rays of approximately 4000 nm
* radiant heat rays which are shorter wavelength rays of approximately 1000 nm.

An infra-red lamp or non-luminous lamp type emits a gentle warmth with a barely detectable glow. The lamp operates at a fairly low temperature so the intensity of the output is also low.

A radiant heat lamp or luminous lamp type emits a more intense heat with a very visible glow. The lamp operates at a much higher temperature with an output of heat radiation and visible light.

Infra-red and radiant heat lamps are used in therapy treatments to warm the tissues and the difference in the wavelengths produces varying effects.

Infra-red rays penetrate the epidermal layer only irritating the cells to release histamine which results in the blood vessels dilating thus generating heat in the tissues. This redness is often termed *hyperaemia* and has a soothing effect as opposed to a stimulating one as the nerve endings are not greatly affected.

Radiant heat rays penetrate into the dermal layers causing immediate dilation of the blood and lymph vessels which forces the fluids away from the skin into the underlying structures producing a deep heat effect.

Types of infra-red equipment

Infra-red and radiant heat lamps normally come in the following forms:

* **Fireclay lamp** – this is basically a wire coil surrounding a clay support with a reflector shield.

Fig. 9.2 *Infra-red heat lamp*

- **Filament lamp** – this is like a large light bulb which also contains a built in reflector shield and is made from red coloured glass. Dimmer devices are added so the intensity of the lamp can be reduced to emit infra-red rays as opposed to radiant heat.
- **Quartz heat lamp** – this type normally contain quartz rods with a heating element inside. (Sometimes seen as old-fashioned bathroom heaters.)

There is a European recommendation that when using high wattage bulbs the cowl, the part that holds the bulb, should be double skinned to allow an outer and an inner space between the bulb and the cowl. This creates a cooling effect as air drawn into the lower ventilating holes or slits warms, rises, and flows out through the upper ventilation holes or slits.

POINTS TO NOTE ▷

- *Infra-red bulbs are generally 250 watts although 300 watt bulbs can also be purchased.*
- *Ultra-violet bulbs are generally 300 watts.*
- *Normal domestic light bulbs vary up to 100 watts.*
- *Infra-red treatments should not be given on the same day as other heat treatments and in particular should not be given in conjunction with ultra-violet treatments.*

General effects of infra-red and radiant heat on the body

Infra-red and radiant heat are used in the therapy clinic as a general heat treatment to help relax the client and to relieve pain and tension. These effects are achieved as:

- Metabolism is speeded up as a result of the increased heat which will ultimately increase the demand for oxygen and nutrients and speed up the excretion of waste and toxins.
- Vasodilation occurs due to the heat on the blood vessels increasing blood circulation.
- Sudoriferous gland activity is increased due to the vasodilation effect (this will bring about further elimination of waste products).
- Soothing effect on sensory nerve endings.

CONTRAINDICATIONS to infra-red and radiant heat treatments

! Heart and vascular conditions.

! Fever, heavy colds and influenza.

! Skin diseases and disorders.

! High or low blood pressure.

! Burns and sunburn.

! Metal pins and plates.

256

! Diabetics (due to impaired circulation).

! Oedema.

! Cuts, scars and skin abrasions.

Harmful effects of infra-red and radiant heat treatment
If the treatment is not carried out correctly any of the following may occur:

* Burning of the skin.
* Giddiness or fainting.
* Headaches.
* Permanent eye injury.

Safety precautions for infra-red and radiant heat treatment

1 Always carry out a detailed consultation before treatment checking for any contraindications.

2 Always follow manufacturer's instructions with regard to operating any equipment.

3 Accurately time and position the lamp according to the cosine and inverse square laws (see below).

4 Protect the client's eyes.

5 Ensure skin is properly prepared and carry out a skin sensitivity test prior to treatment. (See Chapter 6.)

6 Ensure lamp is secure with no trailing wires, is dust free and is regularly serviced.

7 Preheat lamp before positioning over treatment area.

8 Do not leave the client unattended.

PROGRESS CHECK

1 List the key principles of the electromagnetic spectrum.
2 Name the three types of infra-red equipment available.
3 What is the average wattage of an infra-red bulb?
4 List four effects of infra-red/radiant heat.
5 List five contraindications to infra-red and radiant heat treatments.

The cosine law

The cosine law shows the comparison between intensity of rays and the angle at which these rays make contact with the skin. The lamp should be placed perpendicular to the skin ensuring the rays fall at right angles to the body which will give maximum intensity.

With the lamp placed
at right angles the
rays will cover only a
small area

With the lamp placed
at a reduced angle the
rays now cover a larger
area thus reducing the intensity

Fig. 9.3 *The cosine law*

The inverse square law

With any radiation treatment distance is extremely important and in
particular it is important when using ultra-violet where very little heat is
generated. It goes without saying that the closer a lamp is to the body
the higher the intensity of radiation will be. The inverse square law states
that *the intensity of radiation will differ inversely with the square of the distance from
the lamp.* This means that if the distance from the lamp is doubled the
intensity of the rays will be quartered. In practical terms the intensity of
radiation at a distance of 30 cm is four times that at 60 cm, i.e. four
minutes treatment at 60 cm will give the same effect as one minute at
30 cm.

Fig. 9.4 *The inverse square law*

ACTIVITY   Research the uses of infra-red heat treatments within a health spa.

Ultra-violet radiation

Ultra-violet rays have wavelengths within the range of 200 to 400
nanometres, i.e. beyond the violet end of the visible light spectrum. They
are invisible to the naked eye and are classified as follows:

- UVA rays.
- UVB rays.
- UVC rays.

UVA *rays*

UVA rays have wavelengths of 315–400 nm and penetrate deeply into the dermal layer of the skin. This damages the collagen and elastin fibres causing premature ageing together with increasing the risk of skin cancer. UVA rays expand melanin already present within the skin causing a short term tanning effect.

UVB *rays*

UVB rays have wavelengths of 280–315 nm and will penetrate only to the basal layer of the epidermis. UVB stimulates melanocytes present in this layer to produce more melanin causing a much deeper, longer lasting colour than UVA alone. It is UVB which causes thickening of the epidermis and is also responsible for sunburn and for the development of skin cancers.

POINTS TO NOTE ▷

* *If a client chooses or is recommended to have a UVB treatment, a pre-sensitisation and a skin sensitivity test (see Chapter 6) must be carried out in addition to the therapist observing contraindications and safety precautions.*
* *It is paramount that the cosine and inverse square laws are implemented.*

Pre-sensitisation test

This should be carried out 24 hours before the client wishes to have the UVB treatment. One way to carry out such a test is to take a sheet of paper and cut four small holes in a line about 1 cm apart. Place the sheet over the forearm and mount the UV lamp at the standard distance. Expose the area to UV rays for one and a half minutes then cover over the first hole, continue UV exposure and after a further half a minute cover over the second hole, after another half a minute cover the third hole and the final hole after another half a minute. The arm should be

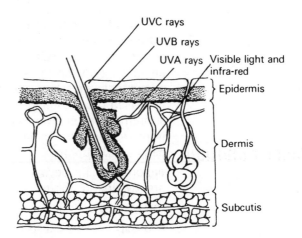

Fig. 9.5 *Ultra-violet and Infra-red penetration of the skin*

inspected the following day to see which of the areas most closely resembles a first degree erythema so the appropriate exposure time can be worked out for the client.

UVC *rays*

UVC rays have a wavelengths shorter than 280 nm and are harmful to living cells. UVC rays are absorbed by the Earth's atmosphere and therefore are not found in natural sunlight or used in salon tanning treatments.

The effects of ultra-violet radiation

Current research into the effects of ultra-violet radiation have proved that it is responsible for premature ageing of the skin together with being the primary cause of skin cancer. In extreme moderation however there are some beneficial effects:

- Stimulates the production of vitamin D needed for healthy bones and teeth.
- Has a slightly germicidal effect on the skin.
- Causes hyperkeratinisation which is thought to help with some skin conditions such as acne vulgaris and psoriasis.
- Gives a psychological feeling of well being.
- Produces a tan.

Harmful effects of ultra-violet treatment

- May cause sunburn if exposure is too long.
- Is the primary cause of skin cancer.
- Thickens the epidermis giving a 'leathery' appearance.
- Irreversibly damages collagen and elastin fibres leading to premature ageing.
- Causes dehydration of the skin tissues.
- Can cause allergic reactions.
- Can produce dark pigmentation patches.

The tanning mechanism

Ultra-violet rays are absorbed by the skin where they stimulate an enzyme called *tyrosinase*, found within the epidermis, which converts into an amino-acid known as *tyrosin* which then changes into *melanin*. This is an immediate response to exposure to ultra-violet and is followed by the increased production of new skin cells which quickly migrate to the stratum corneum layer to develop in colour. Prolonged exposure to UVB in particular will stimulate greater melanocyte production causing a deep and lasting tan.

The way in which this tanning mechanism works will depend on the individual skin type and colouring. These skin types are normally categorised as follows:

- Group 1 – very sensitive, burns easily and never develops a tan.
- Group 2 – sensitive skin which burns easily and tans with difficulty.

* Group 3 – normal skin which tans fairly slowly and may burn slightly.
* Group 4 – tans very easily without burning.
* Group 5 – genetically pigmented skin which rarely burns.

Sunburn

Sunburn is the result of damage to the skin and is the body's way of protecting itself. Sunburn presents as erythema a few hours after exposure. Erythema is the result of histamine being released in the tissues which causes dilation of the blood capillaries. In extreme cases plasma exudes from the blood vessels into the tissues causing blisters.

There are four degrees of erythema which are as follows:

* First degree – presents as slight redness with no irritation and disappears after 24 hours.
* Second degree – presents as a more marked redness with irritation lasting for 2–3 days.
* Third degree – presents as very hot skin which is sore and swollen with pigmentation and lasts for up to one week; desquamation will occur.
* Fourth degree – this is similar to a third degree with the addition of blisters and peeling. This can be quite serious and require medical treatment.

PROGRESS CHECK

1 Briefly explain the relevance of the cosine and inverse square laws.

2 Give the three bands of ultra-violet rays and explain their main effects.

3 State the purpose of the skin sensitivity and pre-sensitisation tests.

4 List the contraindications to ultra-violet treatments.

5 Give five harmful effects of ultra-violet radiation.

6 Briefly outline the stages of tanning.

7 Give a brief description of the four degrees of sunburn.

Types of ultra-violet equipment

Within the beauty salon ultra-violet radiation can be utilised in four ways:

* Mercury vapour lamps.
* Solarium.
* Sun-bed.
* Wood lamp.

Mercury vapour lamps

This type of equipment consists of a lamp surrounded by a layer of quartz which allows UV rays to pass through. The space between contains argon gas and a small amount of mercury. Two electrodes are encased at either end. When the unit is switched on ionisation of the argon gas occurs and electrons flow through the tube; this, together with the ionisation of the mercury, produces ultra-violet radiation. This type of equipment is rarely used in the therapy clinic but can be seen in hospitals for the treatment of certain skin conditions such as psoriasis.

Solarium

These normally consist of a lamp or a group of lamps suspended in an overhead fashion and often combining infra-red bulbs with UVB emitters. Traditionally these were used for either preparing the client's skin for exposure to sunlight by using UVB rays or for preparing the client for further salon treatments such as massage by using the infra-red lamps contained within the unit. Modern technology has seen the development of solarium-type units which encompass a padded bed area and air conditioning together with a small, high-pressure area for the face. Some also include music facilities. Those with infra-red as well as ultra-violet rays generate more heat and thus have a relaxing effect for the client. Individual manufacturer's instructions need to be followed closely to calculate treatment exposure and classify the type of UV rays emitted.

Sun-bed

These are the most popular form of UV equipment seen in the salon today and normally consist of a single or double sided plastic covered bed containing UV tubes. Modern beds are usually contoured to ensure even tanning treatment. The tubes are often made from a product called vita-glass which allows the UV rays to pass through. Vita-glass has a phosphorous lining which absorbs UVC and most UVB rays thereby emitting almost exclusively UVA. At the ends of the sun-bed tube the rating and specification will be stamped. Those with a built-in reflector will be marked R-UVA. Great care must be taken to ensure the correct type of replacement lamp is chosen for each sun-bed.

Note. R-UVA tubes should not be fitted into early models of sun-bed which have reflector panels between each lamp fitting position because a 'striped' tan will result! Check ratings of lamps carefully and consider the overall intensity per bed according to the number of lamps used.

Fig. 9.6 Sunbed

POINTS TO NOTE ▷

* *Always ensure the plastic surfaces have been cleaned between clients using a specific product for the purpose as the wrong type of cleaner can damage them.*
* *Always use the manufacturer's recommended emission tubes and keep detailed records of tube use.*
* *Never leave a client unattended throughout the treatment.*

Wood lamp

Wood lamps can be used to assist the therapist in the analysis of their clients' skin. 'Black' ultra-violet tubes illuminate skin conditions in degrees of reflected light, which gives a far clearer view than the naked eye sees in normal light. A variety of lamps are available; traditionally they are designed to be used in a darkened room. Some incorporate the use of a magnifying lamp and a black-out screen; the most consumer conscious enable the client to view their skin 'illuminated' at the same time as the therapist. An accurate and very visual analysis of their skin condition is very motivating and encourages a client to follow the treatment and home care schedule recommended by their therapist.

Fig. 9.7 *Wood lamp*

Ultra-violet treatment

As with any salon treatment, a detailed consultation should be carried out with the client before using UV equipment. Contraindications and a skin sensitivity and/or pre-sensitisation test should be checked thoroughly.

CONTRAINDICATIONS

to ultra-violet treatments

- **!** Any person who does not tan naturally in the sun.
- **!** Any person prone to frequent bouts of coldsores (herpes simplex).
- **!** Pigmentation disorders; vitiligo, chloasma.
- **!** Vascular problems.
- **!** Migraine and headache suffers.
- **!** Any person prone to fainting.
- **!** Pregnancy (as this may lead to increased pigmentation – chloasma).
- **!** Previous history of skin cancer, problems with moles.
- **!** Fever, colds and high temperature.
- **!** Certain drugs may cause photosensitisation; antibiotics, tranquillisers, diuretics, contraceptive pills, anti-diabetic tablets, cold injections, quinine, blood pressure medications. (Consent from the client's GP will be required in these cases.)

Safety precautions for ultra-violet treatment

If it is considered safe to give treatment the client must:

- Remove all make-up and perfume and ensure that the skin is completely dry.
- Remove watches and jewellery.
- Shower with an unperfumed product.
- Remove contact lenses.
- Cover hair, especially if treated with colours or permanent wave solutions.
- Avoid applying any suntan preparations except those recommended for UV treatments by specialist manufacturers.
- Wear protective goggles at all times.

Check the client's skin type and colouring. Explain all procedures clearly to the client and supervise the treatment at all times. Ensure that high standards of hygiene are maintained in the treatment area and that manufacturers instructions are clearly followed.

GOOD PRACTICE ▷

- *Treatment should be discontinued if the client has any adverse reaction to the treatment.*
- *Accurate records should be kept of all treatments given.*
- *Ideally perspiration during a sun-bed treatment should be minimal. Most beds contain body-cooling fans to reduce sudoriferous gland activity.*
- *It is essential that the sun-bed room has sufficient ventilation.*

ACTIVITY

Research the variety of suntanning equipment available. Compare their cost, size, facilities, durability and cost effectiveness within a salon environment.

PROGRESS CHECK

1 Explain the benefits of using a wood lamp in the salon.
2 State the differences between ultra-violet and infra-red treatments.
3 State the main benefits and uses of infra-red and ultra-violet treatments.
4 List the safety precautions to be observed when carrying out:
  a solarium treatment
  b infra-red treatment.
5 Explain why pressure marks from a sun-bed do not tan.

KEY TERMS

You need to know what these words and phrases mean. Go back through the chapter to find out.

Ultra-violet	Pre-sensitisation	Sunburn
Infra-red	Cosine law	Solarium
Electromagnetic spectrum	Inverse square law	Sun-bed
Radiant heat	Tanning mechanism	Wood lamp

10 Remedial camouflage

After working through this chapter you will be able to:

➤ identify the different conditions that can be treated with camouflage make-up
➤ list the contraindications to camouflage techniques
➤ have knowledge of the basic principles required to carry out treatment
➤ carry out a basic camouflage make-up treatment.

In today's society great emphasis is placed on physical appearance. Whether we like it or not, we are all influenced by media pressure to look the very best that we can even if this is sometimes an unhealthy attitude to possess.

For some this can be made worse by unnatural disfigurement caused either at birth or through illness or accident. While surgery may be an option for some, it is not possible or necessary for others, yet they still feel embarrassment every time they face the outside world. This can have serious repercussions, in some cases making the individual loathe to face anything or anyone new. It can affect career prospects and even the forming of relationships.

The therapist who can provide and instruct on remedial camouflage can greatly enhance an individual's life and gain tremendous job satisfaction.

Fig. 10.1 *Remedial camouflage make-up*

Role of the cosmetic camouflage therapist

It goes without saying that the therapist working in cosmetic camouflage is entering into a field slightly different from the normal course of work, with the exception maybe of electrology. This area of work requires a very discreet approach and a sympathetic attitude so as to prevent the client suffering undue stress or discomfort. The therapist should have a good understanding of the different types of disfigurement possible and be able to identify the client's needs and anticipated outcomes. The experienced therapist should be able to expertly cover any blemishes or disfigurement and most importantly be able to instruct the client on how to do so. This should always be carried out in an atmosphere of peace and tranquillity.

266

Client consultation

The importance of a correct client consultation cannot be overstated if the treatment is ultimately going to be a success. The first objective is to establish a rapport with the client and instil confidence in the therapist's ability and willingness to help whilst at the same time being realistic in the treatment outcomes.

It is wise to try and gather information about the scar/disfigurement at the time of booking the consultation so that a general practitioner's note can be provided ahead of time where necessary. This is preferable to referring the client to her/his GP at the time of consultation as it could possibly lead to lost custom through embarrassment or frustration.

It is also most important to allow the client to tell you what is troubling them rather than just presuming. A wrong assessment could cause untold harm to an already sensitive client and this could have serious long-term repercussions on the individual's self-image.

A detailed record card should be completed carefully with the client. An example of such a record card is shown in Fig. 10.2.

Name of client:	Name of doctor:
Address:	Address:
Telephone: Day	Telephone:
Evening:	
Source of referal:	
Type/age of scarring:	
Area(s) of scarring:	
Signature of client:	Signature of therapist:

Fig. 10.2 *Example of a remedial camouflage consultation card*

On the back of the card the following information should be recorded:

* Products used.
* Shades of creams.
* Number/method of application.
* Results.

A similar card should be given to the client after treatment detailing the products used and the method of application so that it can be used for reference. In some cases it may be necessary to also send a copy of the consultation card to the client's own doctor, especially if consent was required or if there is to be any follow-up medical treatment.

Types of client

Unlike in any other area, the therapist working in remedial camouflage will be dealing with a diverse range of clients; men, women and even children. Some will be new to the clinic, some existing and many will be extremely nervous.

Male approach

Men who come to the clinic for remedial camouflage may often be more inhibited than women. This is partly because they consider salons to be the domain of women, especially if there is a feminine style decor and because they see cosmetics as a predominantly female medium. When dealing with a male client the main objective is to make the remedial camouflage as undetectable as possible and to ensure appropriate surroundings.

Female approach

The female client will often be more used to cosmetics and therefore less inhibited about using them. She may however be more concerned about her appearance than a male client so may need extra reassurance and even help and guidance with normal cosmetic application.

Child approach

When dealing with children for remedial camouflage it is important not to make them feel that their disfigurement is unacceptable. Often it is a parent who has instigated treatment and this can draw attention in the child's mind to a problem that never really bothered them before. Depending on the age of the child it may be a case of teaching the parent how to apply camouflage techniques. It should be suggested that in this case the child returns at a later date to be given expert advice as well.

Also it is worth mentioning that some childhood disfigurements disappear with age in some instances.

PROGRESS CHECK

1 State the importance of the consultation procedure.
2 Explain how you would handle a child requiring cosmetic camouflage.

Remedial camouflage conditions

Pigmentation disorders

The most common pigmentation disorders are outlined here.

Chloasma

This is a smooth, irregularly shaped patch of brown pigmentation which occurs when there is increased production of the melanocyte stimulating hormone. It occurs most frequently in pregnancy or when taking the contraceptive pill. Exposure to ultra-violet radiation exacerbates the condition.

Vitiligo (leucoderma)

This is an absence of melanin in small patches on the skin caused by the destruction of melanocytes in the basal layer of the epidermis. Sometimes large areas can be affected and the small patches merge into one. The condition is obviously more noticeable on a darker skin. The other key feature of vitiligo is that as there is no protective melanin present, the areas affected are photosensitive and will burn if exposed to UV radiation.

Melanoderma

This is a general term for patchy pigmentation of the skin. There are many reasons for melanoderma but the main cause is allergic reaction to a product being applied to the skin and reacting with UV radiation, e.g. perfume.

Types of naevus

The medical definition of a naevus is a birthmark or circumscribed area of pigmentation due to dilated blood vessels. Many forms of naevus exist including;

* Strawberry naevus. These are normally present at birth or occur shortly afterwards and normally start as a small red spot which enlarges fairly quickly. They are normally raised above the surface of the skin and can become quite large. In most cases they fade with time and will have completely disappeared by the age of about seven when just a red patch remains.
* Angioma (Port wine stain). So named because it tends to be dark red or purplish in colour. Angioma can be extremely disfiguring. It is an area of profusely dilated capillaries and often affects the face and neck. The individual is born with this condition.
* Spider naevus (stellate haemangioma). These can appear at any age and are small, red central spots with superficial veins radiating from them. They can occur on any part of the body, but are usually seen on the face and upper cheek area.
* Epidermal benign naevus (moles). Moles can be found all over the body and vary in size and texture. They can be raised or flat, pigmented or normal skin colour, and some contain hairs. Most pigmented moles occur through overgrowth of melanocytes in the basal layer of the epidermis which is an indirect result of exposure to ultra violet radiation.

Types of scar

A scar is a mark which is left on the skin after it has healed from some form of trauma. There are many different types of scarring, but the main categories are outlined here.

Hypertrophic scar

This is a large unsightly scar which is raised and shiny in appearance.

Ice-pick scar

As the name suggests, this type of scar is rough and pitted. It is a common post-acne blemish.

GOOD PRACTICE ▷ *Applying the cosmetics with a brush is excellent for thin, 'hairline' type scars as the cream should not be spread in too large an area.*

Keloid scar

This type of scar is fibrous and lumpy as the body continues to produce extra collagen after a wound has healed. Keloid scars are more prevalent on black skin types.

Quiescent scar tissue

This term describes scar tissue which is at rest or has healed. The rate at which a scar will heal will vary from one person to another. There are general signs that will indicate that a scar is healed:

* there is no evidence of inflammation
* it is not painful or sensitive to the touch
* it is not weeping or moist.

Skin disorders

Psoriasis

This is caused by an abnormally fast rate of cell renewal in the epidermis with cells sometimes reaching the stratum corneum in a few days instead of the normal 28–30. This results in clusters of cells forming characteristic oval, dull-red plaques together with silvery scales.

The cause of the condition is not clear but hereditary factors play an important part and it is thought to be exacerbated by stress.

Rosacea

This normally affects the over thirties age group and often women of menopausal age. It begins with a flushed appearance, particularly in response to stress, spicy foods and alcohol. The flushing then becomes permanent as the blood vessels in the area become dilated. This increases the temperature of the skin stimulating sebum production and this in turn leads to papules, pustules and open pores becoming present. It is a chronic disorder of the blood vessels of the face.

Skin conditions

Tattoos

It has long been fashionable for people to have tattoos. A tattoo is where a permanent pigment is put into the skin. Unfortunately many people live to regret having a tattoo and although removal is now possible it is both painful and expensive. Camouflage make-up is an alternative option to successfully hide such marks.

POINT TO NOTE   *Camouflage make up will generally last longer on dry skin types.*

Varicose veins

Varicose veins produce a characteristic bulging effect and can be quite disfiguring. They are the result of valves within the veins collapsing through an inherited weakness and/or poor circulation.

CONTRAINDICATIONS   to camouflage make-up

As with any treatment there are some conditions that the therapist should not treat. Examples include:

! Infectious skin conditions.

! Warts.

! Cuts/Abrasions.

! Skin irritations.

! Swelling.

PROGRESS CHECK

1 List four contraindications to camouflage make-up and explain why each is a contraindication.

2 Describe four types of scar tissue.

3 Name three remedial camouflage conditions which can be successfully camouflaged.

Equipment required for camouflage make-up

A camouflage make-up kit is needed by the therapist which should be kept in an immaculate and hygienic condition. Firstly it will be necessary to have a range of skin care products to prepare the skin for treatment. The client may already be wearing some form of make-up but if not it is still necessary to cleanse and remove any traces of sweat, sebum and general dirt. Toner must be used to remove any residue left by the cleansing medium otherwise the camouflage creams may 'slide' on application and also be unstable. Moisturiser should also be applied, but avoid the blemished area for the same reasons.

Secondly it will be essential to have a good range of cover creams, there are many different types available and it is up to the individual therapist to decide which range is best for them. Great improvements have been made over recent years in the production of camouflage make-up. Products are easier to apply and blend and produce a light, natural look. Many manufacturers produce sample kits of all the colours in their range with replacements available for the colours that are used the most. It will also be important to carry a range of stock for the client to purchase for immediate use.

Within the kit it will be necessary to have a setting or fixing powder. Some manufacturers supply these powders whilst others recommend the use of translucent powder. Retail powder should also be available for the client to purchase. Finally, a range of sponges and good quality sable brushes together with some form of mixing palette will be needed for professional application. Some of the palettes available today are made

271

Fig. 10.3 'Blend-in' palette

from clear Perspex with a central magnifier which allows the therapist to blend the creams and hold it up to the skin to check the colour compatibility. (An example of this type of palette is the one produced by Rita Roberts.)

Lighting

The source and type of lighting is very important when carrying out a camouflage make-up treatment as it will affect the colour of the cosmetics.

The colour of the pigment within the skin will vary depending on the type of light that is illuminating it. Natural daylight is composed of all the colours of the spectrum and will therefore define the face clearly. Artificial (white) light may consist of many hues (colours) some of which may be stronger than others, therefore if the coloured hue falls on a pigment that is able to reflect it the colour of the lighting is seen, however if it falls onto pigment and the rays are absorbed then the pigment colour will be distorted.

Example. If white light falls on a red lipstick the pigment within the product reflects the red light and absorbs the other six colours of the spectrum making the lipstick appear red. However if pure blue light falls on the lipstick it will be absorbed and as there is no red light for it to reflect it will appear black.

ACTIVITY   **Research the effects of lighting on make-up.**

Camouflage make-up creams

When choosing a range of camouflage make-up it is important to consider the following points:

• Colour range. There should be a wide range of colours available to cater from the palest to the darkest skin colouring.

272

* Even consistency. The products should blend easily on contact with the skin, they should not drag or feel unduly tacky.
* Waterproof. The products should be waterproof to allow the user to participate in normal activities, e.g. swimming.
* UV filters. As scar tissue can be sensitive, cover creams should have in-built UV filters.

Blending techniques

If the therapist is to become skilled in the blending of camouflage make-up it is essential to have a good understanding of the principles of colour and to practise.

The colour wheel

There are three primary colours; red, blue and yellow. To make a colour you move around the wheel, e.g. red + yellow = orange.

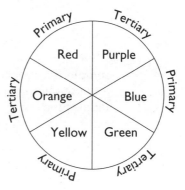

Fig. 10.4 *The colour wheel*

POINT TO NOTE ▷ *Opposite colours neutralise, e.g. green neutralises red.*

Colourings

The colour of skin can alter through life as it is affected by different factors such as climate, illness and certain products.

Skin contains varying amounts of the pigment melanin which is genetically passed from parent to child. Skin colour can be divided into four basic categories

1 Caucasian skin. This is the most fragile of all skin types, prone to sun damage, broken capillaries and pigmentation irregularities. Scarring tends to leave pink pigmentation marks that can be quite noticeable. It has blue and pink tones present from the blood capillaries behind which is a basic tone normally of either yellow or pink. It can vary from being very pale to quite a deep tan depending on UV exposure and hereditary factors.

2 Oriental skin. This type is more resilient than Caucasian skin and most often is of even tone. However it can develop pigmentation discoloration if exposed to ultra violet radiation. This skin type will have more melanin present and be mainly of one colour tone. It has a basic yellow undertone.

3 Asian skin. This type is normally strong and adaptable. It can have a tendency towards uneven colouring and in particular dark shadows around the eye area. Scarring tends to leave dark pigmentation marks which are slow to fade. It can vary in tone from being quite olive to very dark, but always has a yellow undertone.

4 Black skin. This skin type has the greatest amount of protective melanin pigment and therefore is the slowest to show signs of ageing. As with Asian skin types scarring tends to leave dark pigmentation marks that are slow to fade. There are many varying colour tones from light brown to deep ebony.

ACTIVITY

Complete a detailed case study on a client with a disfigurement, keeping photographic evidence where possible. Evaluate your findings including client feedback.

Matching skin colour (basic application techniques)

As mentioned previously, when purchasing a camouflage make-up kit it is essential to choose one with a good variety of depths and tones of shades to meet the diverse range of skin colours.

1 It will be necessary to establish the depth and tone of the client's skin and to chose the nearest colour to match the client's skin accordingly.

2 Neutralise any irregularities present, e.g. green will neutralise red, but it must be remembered that the principle of camouflage make-up is to disguise the abnormality by blending it to the client's skin colour.

3 Mix the depths and tones so that when applied to the treatment area it will blend and match the client's skin colour.

4 When choosing the correct colour, if the client's skin is midway between two shades, blending equal quantities of both should produce the exact match.

5 If a client's skin is closer to one of the shades, blending two parts of the closer to one part of the other should produce a good match.

6 Another important point is to write down exactly what has been blended as it is easy to forget.

Once you have mixed the correct shade it will be necessary to test the cream near the treatment area. If the match is perfect it can be applied to the disfigurement. However if it is deeply pigmented it may not be sufficient to adequately cover, in which case it will be necessary to apply a thin coat then set it with powder and then apply a second coat and set that.

POINT TO NOTE

A dampened cosmetic sponge is used when a light coverage is required. For example a camouflage treatment for rosacea to give a natural look will allow some of the skin's natural colouring to show through.

There are many methods for applying camouflage make-up and whichever method is chosen it will require a lot of practise to become proficient. There are a few basic principles which the therapist should observe;

* Always thoroughly prepare the area before treatment with cleansing, toning and moisturising procedures but avoid putting moisturiser directly over the scar.

* Always study the skin colour and type of disfigurement carefully.

* Always apply camouflage creams sparingly as this will achieve a more natural effect and is less likely to come off on clothing.

* Apply the creams in layers, setting between applications (except where an additional cream is to be added to the basic shade as in the case of toning-in with a surrounding area, in which case the powder is applied at the end).

USEFUL INFORMATION

The finger can be used in several ways; in a rubbing action, a pressing action or in a stippling action. This means that you can control the amount of surface stimulation of the blood capillaries which is very important in certain conditions.

* Always allow a few minutes for the products to set properly and then brush off the powder in a downward action.

* Blot the area gently with damp cotton wool to remove any detectable traces of powder.

* Use either a brush, dampened cosmetic sponge or even a finger to apply cosmetic camouflage depending on size and area of treatment, and always work in a hygienic fashion.

* Use feathering strokes to fade-in the edges around the camouflage area.

* Always explain procedures to the client and give home care advice on general skin care, removal, application at home, etc.

* Ask the client to book in for a further consultation so that any queries can be dealt with and you can see how they are progressing with their application techniques.

GOOD PRACTICE

▷ * *Remember to try and contain the cosmetics to the area requiring camouflage for the most natural effect.*

  * *The appearance of stubble will sometimes need to be added to men and this can be achieved by carefully stippling a grey coloured cream.*

ACTIVITY

With a colleague, practise camouflaging disfigurements such as freckles, scars, birthmarks, etc. Take the role of the client and therapist and carry out a detailed consultation. Evaluate your findings.

Home care advice

1 Camouflage make-up should be removed thoroughly with an appropriate product.

2 Be careful with soap or soap-based products as these can sometimes dislodge the creams.

3 When drying with a towel after bathing or swimming always pat dry and do not rub the camouflaged area.

4 Climate can have an effect on the durability of the products as heat tends to loosen the creams more readily. For this reason a client will need to take great care whilst in any hot environment.

POINT TO NOTE ▷ *Artificial freckles sometimes need to be added to restore balance to the face.*

Prosthetics

This is the term used to describe any manufactured appendage used to enhance or complete the human body. Obvious examples include artificial limbs, but false nails and eyelashes also fall into the category and an understanding of the different prostheses available will be of benefit to the camouflage therapist.

ACTIVITY

Research the types of prostheses available.

PROGRESS CHECK

1 State the main conditions you may encounter in the field of camouflage make-up.

2 Give three important points to consider when selecting camouflage creams.

3 Explain the importance of lighting when carrying out a camouflage make-up treatment.

4 Give four classifications of skin colour and explain two characteristics of each.

KEY TERMS

You need to know what these words and phrases mean. Go back through the chapter to find out.

Cosmetic camouflage
Client consultation
Remedial camouflage conditions

Equipment required for camouflage
Blending techniques
Matching skin colour
Prosthetics

11

Salon administration and related legislation

After working through this chapter you will:
- ➤ have a greater awareness of what is involved in setting up a business
- ➤ recognise the roles and responsibilities of the employment hierarchy
- ➤ be able to identify the important legislative requirements necessary to conduct a successful business.

Beauty therapy is a diverse and exciting career offering many opportunities and working arrangements. There are few professions where so much choice is available. It is essential that the therapist has a good working knowledge of salon administration and related legislation whether they are a junior therapist, manager or self-employed as the success of the salon ultimately depends on efficient working practices.

Different countries have differing legislation governing business practices. This chapter focuses on those business practices in England and Wales and is not intended to be a definitive one, but more of a guide and source of reference.

Forms of business arrangements

Legally all businesses fall into one of the following categories:
- ⊛ Sole trader.
- ⊛ Partnership.
- ⊛ Limited company.
- ⊛ Franchise.
- ⊛ Co-operative.

Sole trader

This is the simplest form of business organisation. One person controls finance and decisions. From a legal point of view there is nothing that needs to be done to set up in business as a sole trader.

Advantages
- ⊛ Easy to set up – no lengthy legal formalities.
- ⊛ Total control of the business.
- ⊛ Immediate decision making.

Fig. 11.1 *The salon*

* Taxed as an individual.
* Should benefit from close relations with suppliers.
* Easy to wind up.

Disadvantages

* Liable for any business losses.
* No legal distinction between the business and personal assets.
* Possible lack of continuity in management if the owner is ill.
* Does not have status.
* Possible lack of finances for expansion.

Partnership

By definition a partnership is when two or more people go into business together without registering as a limited company or a co-operative.

Again this form of business can be set up without legal formalities, but it is not to be recommended as severe disagreements could jeopardise the business. It is much safer to have a formal partnership agreement drawn up detailing the roles and responsibilities of all partners.

Advantages

* A good way to start up a business that requires more capital than one person alone may have.
* Wider range of complementary skills and knowledge.
* Sharing of workload and general pressures of running a business.
* Sharing of any business losses.

Disadvantages

* All partners are responsible for any business debts even if they are caused by the actions of the other(s).
* Legal costs involved in drawing up a partnership agreement.
* Death or bankruptcy of one partner will automatically dissolve the partnership (unless previous arrangements have been made).
* Possible personality clashes can cause problems.

Limited company

A limited company is formed with a minimum of two shareholders, one of whom must be a director. A company secretary must also be appointed but he/she can be an outsider.

This is a company whereby any business debts are limited to the amount put in. Therefore if the business does go bankrupt, personal possessions cannot be taken to pay the company's debts.

A limited company prior to registration must produce and adhere to two legal documents:

* Memorandum of Association – this sets out the objectives of the company, as well as the company's share capital.
* Articles of Association – sets out additional rules by which the company will be governed.

Advantages

* Limited liability.
* Capital may be increased by selling shares.
* Better definition of management structures.
* Business not affected by death or bankruptcy of any of its shareholders.
* Higher level of status.
* Shareholders are employees of the company and therefore entitled to DSS benefits should the need arise.

Disadvantages

* Costly to set up with time-consuming legal formalities.
* The business will have to make public its accounts.
* As an employee of the company you will be subject to PAYE (see p. 295).

Franchise

A franchise is a business relationship between a franchiser (the owner of a name or method of business) and a franchisee (an operator of that business). The franchisee agrees to pay the franchiser a sum of money for the use of the business name, method of doing business, etc. Often there is an initial fee and an agreed percentage of sales afterwards is paid to the franchiser by the franchisee.

Advantages

* A tried and tested formula.
* A corporate image, instantly recognisable.
* Normally there is a wealth of knowledge available concerning most aspects of the business.
* Back-up services normally provided.
* Sharing of advertising costs.

Disadvantages

* Normally very expensive to set up.
* Business never truly your own.
* Franchiser may lay down certain requirements.
* May not be a flexible enough system to cater for changing needs of a local market.
* Profits normally have to be shared with the franchiser.

Co-operative

A co-operative is a business that is owned and controlled by the people working in it, therefore membership is usually open to all employees. The profits are not shared on the amount of capital put into the business by each individual but are distributed in proportion to the amount of work done by each person.

Choice and type of premises

When setting up in business one of the first things you will need to think about are premises. The type and location of the premises are extremely important and it will be essential to thoroughly research this. Firstly you will need to establish that there is going to be a suitable potential market where you are looking. Local competitors will also need to be taken into account as will parking facilities and neighbouring businesses (you hardly want to be situated next door to a betting office!). If the premises you are interested in are not already occupied as a salon you will need to apply to the local council for a change of use.

POINT TO NOTE ▷ *Never agree to take on premises until you have been granted a change of use.*

You then need to decide whether you are going to buy or rent premises. It will probably be the case that finances dictate your ultimate choice, but remember that sometimes large shopping complexes are owned by large companies or councils so the choice may be taken further from you.

Buying

If you decide that you are going to buy your premises you will need to contact a solicitor immediately to deal with the contracts involved and also to organise a land search. This is to check the ownership of the property and any plans in the future for redevelopment, etc. You will also need to establish if the property is freehold which means that the land and building would be yours if you purchased it, or whether it is leasehold which would mean that the building would be yours but the land that it is built on belongs to a third party and you would need to pay a ground rent.

Renting

Renting, or leasing as it is correctly known, is when you agree to occupy a building in return for an agreed sum of money. If you decide to rent a property you will again need the services of a solicitor to draw up a lease agreement which should include the following:

* How much rent is to be paid and how often (monthly, quarterly, etc.).
* When the amount of rent paid will be reviewed.
* How long the lease will run for.
* Who will be responsible for repairs, upkeep and decoration of the premises both internally and externally.
* What the rules are regarding subletting.
* Awareness of the Landlord and Tenant Act 1954.

Altering premises

Whether you are the owner of the property or just leasing, if you wish to alter the premises you will need to check the following:

* Planning permission.

* Building and fire regulations.
* Offices, Shops and Railway Premises Act 1963.

POINT TO NOTE ▷ *Before setting up in business it is essential to prepare a plan, particularly if financial support is needed. Most banks and financial institutions offer guidance and support for small businesses. A business plan should include:*

* *Personal details.*
* *Type of business.*
* *Background of the business, e.g. staff, outgoings, etc.*
* *Products/services.*
* *Business market.*
* *Financial considerations/projections.*
* *Anticipated profits over a number of years.*

PROGRESS CHECK

1 **a** List four forms of business arrangement.
  b Give two advantages and two disadvantages of each form of business arrangement.
2 State four important points to consider when looking for business premises.
3 Compare and contrast buying and renting as an option when deciding on business premises.

Basic business legislation

The Landlord and Tenant Act 1954

This piece of legislation gives the tenant security of tenure which means that you cannot be removed from the premises you are leasing unless the landlord can show a justified reason (not paying the rent, etc.). If the landlord wishes to remove you to sell the premises you will be entitled to compensation.

Offices, Shops and Railway Premises Act 1963

This piece of legislation relates in particular to hygiene, health and safety of the premises and covers such things as:

* Washing facilities.
* Toilets for both sexes and for client use.
* Sanitation.
* Safety on stairways.
* Eating and drinking facilities for staff required to stay on the premises at break-times.
* Adequate space for each employee (at least 400 cubic feet if the ceiling is 10 ft high).
* Fire exits and adequate fire fighting equipment.

Health and Safety at Work Act 1974

This piece of legislation gives rights to both employers and employees.

Employers must provide:

* A safe and healthy workplace.
* Proper safety procedures, e.g. fire exits, etc.
* Safe equipment which is regularly serviced.
* Adequate training to all staff in safety procedures.
* Access to a health and safety policy.

Employees must:

* Follow health and safety procedures.
* Act to protect themselves and others.
* Treat all equipment properly and report any faults.

Electricity at Work Regulations Act 1990

This piece of legislation states that all pieces of electrical equipment in the workplace should be checked annually by a qualified electrician. In particular you should discontinue using any equipment that is broken or damaged, displays exposed wires or worn flexes, has a cracked or broken plug and you should never overload sockets.

Fire Precautions Act 1971

This piece of legislation states that all employees should be trained and aware of emergency fire evacuation procedures. This should include knowledge of the following points:

* Awareness of the nearest fire exit (this should remain unlocked during working time).
* Appropriate assembly point once evacuated.
* Never use lifts in the case of a fire.
* Close all windows and doors on leaving the premises where possible.
* Leave all personal belongings behind.
* Awareness of the location and type of fire fighting equipment available on the premises.

POINT TO NOTE ▷ *Fire fighting equipment checklist*

Extinguisher	Type of fire
Blue (dry powder)	All types
Red (water)	Solid material
Black (carbon dioxide)	Electrical
Green (halon gas)	Electrical
Cream (foam)	Liquids

Control Of Substances Hazardous to He[...] 1988

These regulations lay down the ways in which su[...] deemed hazardous to health (for example hydrogen [...] used and stored.

All employees should be made aware of the risks of such sub[...] where necessary be given further training in such areas.

Detailed instructions must be kept regarding any products conside[...] hazardous.

ACTIVITY	Research the symbols used for substances hazardous to health.

The Sale of Goods Act 1979

This act relates to all goods including food regardless of where purchased. Terms under the act include goods being:

* of merchantable quality, i.e. fit for the purpose for which they are intended
* as stated, for example if a vacuum suction machine is sold with 5 ventouses then they must be included.

Supply of Goods and Services Act 1982

This act was passed to extend the protection given to consumers under The Sale of Goods Act to the provision of services, goods on hire and goods given in exchange for vouchers. A client disappointed with a beauty treatment could take action against the salon if it was proved that reasonable care had not been taken under the terms of the Supply of Goods and Services Act

Trade Descriptions Act 1968 and 1972

This act makes it a criminal offence to describe goods falsely, and to sell or offer for sale goods which have been so described. It covers many things including advertisements, display cards, oral descriptions and applies to quality, quantity, fitness for purpose and price. The part of the act passed in 1972 deals with labelling of the country of origin; a product must be clearly labelled so that the consumer can see where it was made.

The Sex Discrimination Acts 1975 and 1986 and The Race Relations Act 1976

The aims of these acts are to prevent direct or indirect discrimination against candidates when applying for work on the grounds of race, sex, or marital status. The Equal Opportunities Commission will investigate complaints made on any of the above grounds and it monitors job advertisements as well.

dismissal – The Employment Protection (Consolidation Act)

piece of legislation identifies situations where it is unfair to dismiss
nployee. Key terms include where an employee is dismissed
use of:

- ining a trade union
- ecting to stay out of a union
- ender or race
- becoming pregnant (but satisfies non-dismissal grounds).

ontract of employment

his is a legally binding document drawn up by the employer when a new
member of staff is appointed. The reason for such a document is to give
both the employer and the employee a certain degree of protection and
security and to formalise specific points. By law any person working 16
hours or more a week must be given a contract of employment within 13
weeks of the starting date.

The contract should cover the following points;

- Name of the company and the employee.
- Date when employment began.
- Job description.
- Hours of work.
- Pay scale, how payment will be made and at what intervals (weekly, monthly, etc.).
- Holiday entitlement.
- Pension arrangements.
- Sickness and sick pay conditions.
- Length of notice which an employee is entitled to give and receive.
- Disciplinary procedures.

There are other conditions which may be added such as working at
different locations, confidentiality, medical examinations, etc. and these
are sometimes presented in a separate staff handbook.

Maternity rights

In England and Wales, women employees who satisfy the relevant
qualifying conditions are entitled to the following statutory rights;

- Paid time off to receive ante-natal care. A woman who is advised by a properly qualified person to attend an ante-natal clinic has the right not to be unreasonably refused time off during her working hours to enable her to keep an appointment.
- Protection from dismissal by reason of pregnancy. A woman with the necessary length of employment is automatically held to be unfairly dismissed if the reason or principal reason for the dismissal is either that she is pregnant or any other reason connected with the pregnancy.

284

USEFUL INFORMATION

Certain local authorities recommend exemption of fees relating to local bye-laws for members of recognised professional bodies considered by them to be health practitioners, e.g. BABTAC.

* Maternity pay. This is currently payable for eighteen weeks to a woman absent from work because of her pregnancy. There are certain qualifying requirements however.
* Return to work after confinement. A woman can currently return to work at any time before the end of the period of twenty nine weeks beginning with the week in which the date of confinement falls.

Local bye-laws concerning body massage treatments

Anyone wishing to set up a clinic offering body massage treatments will probably need a license to practise which is obtained from the local or national licensing authorities. In England and Wales licensing is controlled by the local authority. To qualify for such a license the applicant normally submits information concerning their premises, staff and qualifications. Inspection of the premises is then carried out and once approved by the authority an annual fee is paid which may vary from authority to authority.

Insurance

Insurance is a way of protecting people and property against unforeseen circumstances. It is possible to insure against almost any risk for a sum of money called a premium. In return for this payment, should the risk which you are insuring against occur you will receive compensation to indemnify you for the loss (to be put back in the position you were in before the loss).

When operating in a business certain forms of insurance are compulsory by law. They are as follows:

Public liability insurance

This insurance covers claims relating to injury, disease or damage to the property of a third party (the client). It can be extended to cover liability arising out of goods sold or supplied or if the business involves work away from the premises.

Many professional beauty therapy organisations can arrange group cover which is normally included in some form of membership fee which will generally encompasses other benefits. It is sensible to look at having a one million pound cover against any injury arising out of the treatments offered.

Employers liability insurance

Any business employing staff is legally obliged to have this form of insurance. If an employee is injured at work it is normally the employer who is held responsible whether personally at fault or not. The insurance certificate must be prominently displayed. Any injuries that do occur must be recorded in an accident book.

Although not compulsory by law it is sensible to have insurance to cover:
* Theft.
* Damage to premises, stock and equipment by fire, flood, etc.
* Loss of profits through damage to premises.

- Fidelity bonding (insurance cover to protect against the dishonesty of employees).
- Personal accident insurance.
- Life assurance.

ACTIVITY	Draft a plan of a salon layout, decide on the type of establishment and the number of staff to be employed. Pay particular attention to health, safety, hygiene and legislation.

Staff and recruitment

Role of the employer

The employer has overall control of the well being and efficient running of the business whether or not they are directly involved in it.

Role of the manager/manageress

In smaller establishments this role may be performed by the employer. It is not an easy task requiring a great deal of skill and judgement.

The personal qualities that make a good manager are:

- Enthusiasm about the business and the industry in general.
- Willingness to listen and learn
- Ability to juggle many tasks at the same time; clients, staff, book keeping, wages, etc.
- Patience and tact in dealing with both staff and client problems both on a business and a personal level.
- Knowledge of new trends, e.g. attending exhibitions, reading trade journals, etc.
- Excellent personal and interpersonal skills (tact, diplomacy, punctuality, good communicator, working as a member of a team).
- Immaculate appearance.

The role of the therapist

It goes without saying that the therapist should be well trained and qualified. The therapist needs to be enthusiastic about their work and have a willingness to learn and develop skills. The therapist needs to have a flexible approach and be happy to work as a member of a team, sometimes performing different roles. Again, they should possess excellent personal and interpersonal skills and be of immaculate appearance.

Role of the receptionist

The receptionist is the first point of contact with the salon and therefore an extremely important for the business. The reception area may be staffed by more than one person in larger establishments and by the therapists themselves in smaller concerns. Whoever performs the task needs to be well trained in the workings of the reception area as potential business can be lost through incompetence. (See Chapter 3.)

Support staff

In larger establishments, roles such as cleaning, laundry, handling of stock, preparation of working areas, etc. may be performed by support staff which will obviously add to the overall efficiency of services provided. However it is important that everyone in the establishment can deal with these areas if continuity is to be maintained.

Efficient staff practices

Communication

If the salon is ultimately going to be a successful business it will depend upon efficient levels of communication between all employees thus making the staff more highly motivated and providing a friendly atmosphere for the client.

* Regular staff meetings should be arranged so all employees know what is happening and are allowed to give comments and express their views.
* Staff should be made to feel that they are an important part of the business.
* Staff should be rewarded for anything they do well.
* All employees should be treated equally and fairly.
* Gossip should be discouraged either about clients or fellow employees.
* All employees should be treated with respect.

Staff development

The success of the business lies in expansion and not remaining static. New treatments and ideas should be periodically introduced to increase profit margins, attract new clients and to keep abreast of changes. Staff should be regularly sent on training courses whether they be product knowledge, new skills or further qualifications. This will also help to ensure a highly motivated workforce boosting staff morale.

Appraisal

Appraisal is the term given to a review of an employee's performance over a given period of time, normally annually. The main reason for operating an appraisal system is to help the employee become more effective.

The appraisal is normally categorised into the following areas;

* Review. Looking back over the period concerned, what is the appraisee's job? Has it altered in any way? Is it being performed effectively? Are there any problems?
* Action. What needs to be done? Should there be any training and development? Does the employee need more support/guidance?
* Monitoring. Are the actions being carried out? Are targets being achieved?

POINT TO NOTE ▷ *Ultimately appraisal should be a positive system allowing both the employee and the employer to develop a better understanding of one another. It should lead to increased motivation and provide a basis for reward where it may otherwise be difficult as in the case of commission, etc.*

Costing of treatments

Many salons do not properly cost out their services so therefore they do not make an adequate profit and wonder why the business is not doing very well even though the appointment book is always full. Costing is very important and should encompass materials, overheads, wages and a profit margin.

The following shows an example of a back massage treatment with an explanation underneath;

Back massage treatment (30 minutes)   £12.00

Materials   £1.00

Electricity   £0.60

Laundry   £0.90

Overheads   £1.50

Labour   £4.00

Profit @ 50%   £4.00

* The figures for the materials used are obtained by dividing how much the product would cost at retail by the number of times you can use that product.
* The electricity and overheads costs are calculated by taking the quarterly bills, dividing to find the hourly rate and then dividing again by the number of therapists.
* Laundry is calculated in the same way.
* Labour in this incidence is calculated on the therapist working for £8.00 per hour.
* Profit is calculated on 50% of the total other costs.

PROGRESS CHECK

1 Identify the important legislative requirements necessary to conduct a successful business.

2 What is the main purpose of a contract of employment? Outline the important points such a contract should cover.

3 State the roles and responsibilities of:
   a the employer
   b the manager
   c the therapist
   d the receptionist.

4 What do you understand by the term 'appraisal'?

| ACTIVITY | Cost out a range of salon services based on the example given. |

Marketing and promotion

Many salon owners may wonder why business is not better when they feel they are offering an excellent service, using top quality products and employing well qualified and highly competent staff. The answer probably lies in the fact that they are not marketing themselves sufficiently.

Marketing is not just about placing an advertisement in the local paper, it is the whole product, the image that the salon wishes to create. In the business of aesthetics this is never more important, attention to detail counts. Marketing your services and appropriate skin care products to the right audience requires foresight, empathy, knowledge, enthusiasm and above all, understanding.

Selling in the salon

Selling is a very important aspect of salon operations. Profits made on the sales of products and services make the business successful which will ultimately increase the earning potential of all the employees.

It is important to have a thorough understanding of all the products and treatments available in the salon. Many skin care companies offer product knowledge workshops to familiarise the therapist with the products and methods they offer. If this is not available then it will be essential to read all the information available about the products you intend to sell.

Advice for successful selling

1 Find out exactly what the client needs. This means asking questions and listening carefully to the answers. Use 'closed' questions to get short, straightforward answers (usually yes or no); these help to confirm or eliminate information and ideas. Use 'open' questions to invite fuller and more detailed answers. Open questions help to develop the conversation and provide more personal information.

2 Give the client advice. Always relate the benefits of the product specifically to the client.

3 Always smile and talk confidently and positively about the product which you have chosen. Where possible tell the client about your personal experiences with the product.

4 Explain how the product should be used. If possible let the client feel, smell or hold the product. Remember that if the client touches the product and asks the price, then the item is practically sold.

5 Close the sale. Look for signals that tell you the client has decided to take your advice and buy the product; head nodding in agreement, smiles and friendly eye contact are positive buying signals.

6 Where appropriate, explain the benefits of the different sizes available in the product. These will usually be linked to the price.

Hesitation or reluctance to mention the price will give the client the impression that you consider the product too expensive.

7 Gain agreement with the client. This is achieved either immediately or after a short period of 'thinking' time. Do not be afraid of silences at this stage. Just keep quiet and wait patiently for the client to make a decision. Do not talk yourself out of a sale.

8 Use link selling to encourage your client to buy complementary products from the same range, e.g. cleansers and toners, body exfoliants and lotions, etc.

9 Once you have sold the product, wrap it up and process the payment. As you hand over the purchase, check once more that the client understands how to use the product.

10 Enter the details of the purchase on the client's record card and be sure to ask next time how the client is finding the product.

ACTIVITY	Produce a treatment plan suitable for a client going on a summer holiday, and design a promotional leaflet for the plan

Sales and selling pointers

- Offer samples where possible – most people like to try a product before they buy it and if it is good they will be back to buy.
- Introduce a friend to the salon scheme – if a regular client introduces a friend both should be given some incentive such as a slight discount or a gift, etc.
- Acknowledge all clients' birthdays – in the month of their birthday send each client an incentive to visit the salon.
- Organise new treatment promotions.
- Have new treatment information printed and hand it out to every client.
- Offer special treatment packages – holidays, Christmas, etc.
- Change display areas very regularly.
- Change salon price lists yearly and date them.
- Change salon decor regularly.
- Set out to promote a product every week knowing all its benefits, effects and ingredients (you will soon know your whole range very thoroughly).
- Organise a salon anniversary promotion yearly inviting local press along.
- Make a feature out of a 'slow' day of the week – give it a name and offer extra incentives when people have an appointment on that day.
- Change your own image regularly.

Taxation

Tax can be defined as a compulsory financial contribution imposed by the government in order to raise revenue to support the public services that are used and shared by everyone. There are many forms of taxation – on individual earnings, on the profits of a business, Value Added Tax (VAT) and National Insurance (NI). VAT and NI are explained briefly below.

Value Added Tax (VAT)

This is a tax that is levied by the Government on most business transactions known as 'taxable supplies'. If a business has a taxable turnover greater than £46,000 (current level) it must register for VAT, filling out the appropriate form from the VAT office. A registration number will then be issued and detailed records will need to be kept of all business transactions. The salon owner will need to charge VAT on services provided and products sold, currently standing at 17.5%, and will be liable to pay VAT on equipment and products purchased from VAT registered companies. These are referred to as outputs and inputs respectively. Every three months (VAT tax period) it will be necessary to fill in a form known as a VAT return. Where output tax exceeds input tax the difference will need to be paid to customs and excise, and the reverse where input tax is greater than the output - then it may be reclaimed from customs and excise.

POINT TO NOTE ▷ *The Government has the right to decide which products/services are liable to VAT charges. Those which are not are referred to as* zero *rated examples which include books, newspapers, drugs, children's clothing and footwear.*

National Insurance contributions

This is a tax paid by every working person to the inland revenue to support public services, the unemployed and to help towards the payment of a pension in old age. They should be collected by the employer in the case of employees. There are five classes of National Insurance contribution;

- **Class 1.** These are contributions for employed persons.
- **Class 1a.** These are contributions paid when your employer provides you with a car.
- **Class 2.** These are contributions to be paid by the self-employed. They can be paid either by direct debit through a bank or by stamping a card. If earnings fall below the *lower earnings limit* it may be possible to apply for exemption, but entitlement to some of the benefits provided may be lost.
- **Class 3.** These are voluntary contributions.
- **Class 4.** These are additional contributions that may be made by the self-employed person and are calculated on the profits of the business.

(More information on NI is available from your local inland revenue office.)

Basic business terminology

Insolvency

This is a term used to describe either a business or a person who is unable to pay their debts (bankrupt).

Liquidation

This refers to the winding up of a business to pay off its debts.

Professional standards (ethics)

Every profession has a code of conduct and beauty therapy is no exception. The code stipulates how the therapist should conduct him/ herself in order to obtain a high professional standard.

Medical problems

* Do not carry out any medical treatments.
* Do not give injections.
* Do not cut or sever the skin in any way.
* Do not prescribe oral medication.
* Never treat a client under a doctor's care without obtaining written permission.
* Do not criticise any treatment being given by a doctor.
* Always refer to a doctor if you think a client has a medical problem.
* Try to foster good relations with your local medical practitioners.

Salon manners

* Do not enter into discussions on sex, religion, politics or any other potentially controversial subjects with your clients.
* Never discuss one client with another.
* Do not repeat information you have been told in confidence.
* Avoid repeating bad publicity about other therapists or salons.
* Do not act in a manner that may bring the profession into disrepute.

Advertising

* Never make false claims.
* Do not practise undercutting of prices.
* Do not compare yourself in advertisements with other salons.

Banking

Bank statement

A bank statement is document issued by a bank to all account holders normally on a monthly basis showing all the transactions that have occurred for that period. It will detail how much money is in the account, how much has been put in and taken out.

Cash flow

This can be defined as the flow of money in and out of a business. A cash flow statement is compulsory for all large companies.

EXAMPLE OF A CASH FLOW FORECAST   from ___19___ to ___19___

Period (e.g. 4 weeks/Month/Quarter												
	Budget	Actual	Budget	Actual	Budget	Actual	Budget	Actual	Budget	Actual	Budget	Actual
ORDERS												
SALES												
PURCHASES												
RECEIPTS:												
Sales – cash												
– debtors												
Loans/Grants Received												
Capital Injected												
Asset Disposals												
Other Income												
TOTAL RECEIPTS (CR)												
PAYMENTS:												
Purchases – cash												
– creditors												
Wages, salaries, PAYE												
Rent, rates												
Light, heat, power												
Insurance												
Transport												
Maintenance												
Advertising												
Telephone												
Postage, packaging												
Professional fees												
VAT (net)												
HP payments/leasing charges												
Bank/finance charges and interest												
Loan repayments												
Tax												
Capital Expenditure												
Sundry expenses												
TOTAL PAYMENTS (DR)												
NET CASHFLOW	CR												
	DR												
OPENING BANK BALANCE/ BALANCE BROUGHT FORWARD	CR												
	DR												
CLOSING BANK BALANCE	CR												
	DR												

Fig. 11.2 *Cash flow forecast*

Cheque guarantee card

This card will be requested every time you write a cheque as it is a guarantee to the retailer that the bank will honour the cheque to the value shown on the card. If the card limit is for £50.00 then the bank will only honour a cheque drawn to that amount or less.

Credit card

Credit cards offer a method of paying for goods and services without cash. It can be used as a form of credit (in which case interest will be paid) or the amount can be paid off monthly. A statement of account will be sent out detailing exactly how much you have spent each month.

Current account

This is a bank account that traditionally does not pay interest on any money deposited within it but does give the recipient a cheque book and cheque guarantee card to draw off the account.

Deposit account

This is a bank account that pays interest on any monies deposited in it. There may be clauses attached as to how much notice needs to be given for withdrawals without forfeiting interest.

Standing order

A method of paying for regular expenditures such as a bills. The bank will ask you to fill in a form detailing the person to whom payment is to be made, their bank details and the amount payable. This amount will then be deducted on a regular basis until the bank is notified otherwise.

Direct debit

This is similar to a standing order only this time it is the person requesting the money who instructs the bank to deduct from your account. You will need to fill out a mandate sanctioning the request. Direct debit is very useful where the sum involved may change monthly.

Overdraft

The account holder and the bank agree a limit to which the account may be overdrawn giving a flexible form of finance. Interest will be paid on amount borrowed.

Loan

A formal arrangement with a bank or financial institution allowing an agreed sum of money to be lent to the account holder for an agreed period of time. This is normally for a longer period than an overdraft.

ACTIVITY

Collect information from banks and other financial institutions on the services they offer.

Orders

Advice note

This is a document sent by the supplier to advise when goods will be delivered.

Credit note

This is given by a supplier in exchange for faulty goods and is normally offset against the next invoice.

Delivery note

This document (which is often produced in triplicate) is issued when goods have been ordered and are packed ready for delivery itemising every product. When the driver delivers the goods you are asked to sign the document to confirm that you have received them. One copy is normally given to you, one retained by the supplier and one by the driver.

Pro-forma invoice

This document is issued in particular for a new customer when their credit worthiness is not yet known. It requests payment for goods before they are dispatched.

Book keeping

When setting up in business it will be necessary to keep records of every transaction in a detailed and formal way. The reasons for this are firstly to have documentation of the business's financial position and secondly to allow for an interpretation of the results. It is important to be able to ascertain why things may not be going to well and respond to them.

Whilst it is possible to buy 'off the shelf' book keeping systems, many people who are not expert in the field contract the work out to specialists.

Balance sheet

This is a statement detailing all the assets and liabilities of a business.

Cash book

This book is used to record all payments and receipts carried out on a daily basis together with what has been paid into and taken out of the bank account. It should be periodically checked against bank statements.

Gross profit

This is the term used to describe all profit made before necessary deductions have been taken off.

Net profit

This is a term used to describe the final profit made after all necessary deductions have been made.

PAYE

PAYE stands for 'pay as you earn'. PAYE is applicable to all employees who earn over a specific limit as decided by the government. Earnings related tax and national insurance contributions are deducted under the scheme by the employer.

Petty cash book

A book to record all minor cash transactions including the date, the amount of cash used and the purpose of the transaction.

Profit and loss account
This document summarises all business transactions for a given period (normally one year).

Purchase day book
This allows you to keep a record of any monies that you owe concerning purchases. It should also detail when goods were supplied and the date by which they must be paid for.

Wages book
This is a record of wage/salary details of every employee and will often include personnel information such as NI number, PAYE number, pension and other deductions.

ACTIVITY

Examine a successful business in your area and try to define the reasons why they have become successful.

PROGRESS CHECK

1 Explain the importance of marketing and promotion in the salon.
2 What do you understand by the term 'value added tax'?
3 List the key principles involved in setting up a business.

KEY TERMS

You need to know what these words and phrases mean. Go back through the chapter to find out.

Forms of business arrangement
Choice and type of premises
Basic business legislation
Staff and recruitment

Marketing and promotion
Taxation
Basic business terminology

Bibliography and further reading

YMCA *Guide to Exercise to Music*, Rodney Cullum and Lesley Mowbray, YMCA.

Fitness Leader's Handbook, B. Don Franks and Edward T. Howley

Sear's Anatomy and Physiology for Nurses, R. S. Winwood and J. L. Smith, Edward Arnold.

The Beauty Salon and its Equipment, John V. Simmons, Heinemann.

A Textbook of Anatomy and Physiology, 2nd Ed., W. E. Arnould-Taylor, Stanley Thornes (Publishers) Ltd.

A Practical Guide to Beauty Therapy, Janet Simms, Stanley Thornes (Publishers) Ltd.

Advanced Human Biology, J. Simpkins and J. J. Williams, Collins Educational.

Baillière's Nurses Dictionary, Kasner and Tindall, Baillière Tindall.

GNVQ *Advanced Business*, Roger Lewis and Roger Trevitt, Stanley Thornes (Publishers) Ltd.

Gray's Anatomy, Henry Gray FRS, Senate.

Index

SCOTTISHPOWER TOKEN
EL MEXICANO
EDINBURGH
PLEASE KEEP THIS RECEIPT

POWERCARD
9826 2011 1679 5041 136
0000   POWERCARD
                        KEYED

SALE (MAN)
MOP
                        £5.00
M8045   CASH